PTSD

JOHNS HOPKINS BIOGRAPHIES OF DISEASE
Charles E. Rosenberg, Series Editor

Randall M. Packard, *The Making of a Tropical Disease:
A Short History of Malaria*

Steven J. Peitzman, *Dropsy, Dialysis, Transplant:
A Short History of Failing Kidneys*

David Healy, *Mania: A Short History of Bipolar Disorder*

Susan D. Jones, *Death in a Small Package:
A Short History of Anthrax*

Allan V. Horwitz, *Anxiety: A Short History*

Diane B. Paul and Jeffrey P. Brosco, *The PKU Paradox:
A Short History of a Genetic Disease*

Gerald N. Grob, *Aging Bones: A Short History of Osteoporosis*

Christopher Hamlin, *More Than Hot: A Short History of Fever*

Warwick Anderson and Ian R. Mackay, *Intolerant Bodies:
A Short History of Autoimmunity*

PTSD

❖ ❖ ❖

A Short History

Allan V. Horwitz

JOHNS HOPKINS UNIVERSITY PRESS
Baltimore

2 4 6 8 9 7 5 3

Johns Hopkins University Press
2715 North Charles Street
Baltimore, Maryland 21218-4363
www.press.jhu.edu

Library of Congress Cataloging-in-Publication Data
Names: Horwitz, Allan V., author.
Title: PTSD : a short history / Allan V. Horwitz.
Description: Baltimore : Johns Hopkins University Press, 2018. |
Series: Johns Hopkins biographies of disease | Includes bibliographical
references and index.
Identifiers: LCCN 2017058441 | ISBN 9781421426396 (pbk. : alk. paper) |
ISBN 1421426390 (pbk. : alk. paper) | ISBN 9781421426402 (electronic) |
ISBN 1421426404 (electronic)
Subjects: | MESH: Stress Disorders, Post-Traumatic—history
Classification: LCC RC552.P67 | NLM WM 11.1 | DDC 616.85/21—dc23
LC record available at https://lccn.loc.gov/2017058441

A catalog record for this book is available from the British Library.

*Special discounts are available for bulk purchases of this book. For more information,
please contact Special Sales at 410-516-6936 or specialsales@press.jhu.edu.*

Johns Hopkins University Press uses environmentally friendly book materials,
including recycled text paper that is composed of at least 30 percent
post-consumer waste, whenever possible.

To Esme, Georgia, and Jack

CONTENTS

Foreword, by Charles E. Rosenberg ix
Preface xiii

Chapter 1. A Disorder through Time 1

Chapter 2. PTSD Emerges 19

Chapter 3. The Psychic Wounds of Combat 51

Chapter 4. Diagnosing PTSD 80

Chapter 5. The Return of the Repressed 107

Chapter 6. PTSD Becomes Ubiquitous 135

Chapter 7. Implications 165

Notes 189
Index 231

Disease is a fundamental aspect of the human condition. Ancient bones tell us that pathological processes are older than humankind's written records, and sickness still confounds our generation's newly confident technological capacities. We have not banished pain, disability, or the fear of death even if we die, on average, at older ages, of chronic and not acute ills, in hospital or hospice beds, and not in our own homes. Disease is something men and women feel. It is something in our bodies, but also in our minds—and culture. Disease demands explanation; we think about it and we think with it. Why have I become ill? And why now? How is my body different in sickness from its unobtrusive and uncommunicative functioning in health? What is there about our way of life that might promote endemic ills? Why in time of epidemic has a whole community been scourged?

Answers to such timeless questions necessarily mirror and incorporate available time- and place-specific ideas and assumptions. In this sense, disease has always been a social and linguistic as well as a biological entity. In the Hippocratic era, physicians—and we have always had them with us—were limited to the evidence of their senses in diagnosing a fever, an abnormal discharge, or seizures. But such felt and observable pathologies had to be explained. Classical notions of the somatic basis for such alarming symptoms necessarily reflected and expressed contemporary philosophical and physiological notions, a world of disordered humors and "breath." Today we can call for understanding upon a variety of scientific insights and an ever-increasing armory of diagnostic and therapeutic practices—tools that allow us to diagnose a rich variety of ailments often unfelt by patients and imperceptible to the doctor's senses. In the past century disease has also become an increasingly bureaucratic phenomenon, as sickness has been defined and in that sense partially constituted by formal disease classifications, treatment protocols, and laboratory thresholds.

Sickness is also shaped by ecological realities. How and where we live and how we produce and distribute our resources all contribute to time- and place-specific incidences of disease. For example, ailments such as typhus fever, plague, malaria, dengue, and yellow fever reflect specific environments that we have shared with our insect contemporaries. And humankind's changing physical circumstances are determined in part by culture, especially agricultural practice; disease is thus historically as much as biologically specific. Or perhaps I should say that every disease has a unique past. Once discerned, named, and agreed upon, every disease claims its own history. In this sense, some diseases, such as smallpox or malaria, have a long history; others, like AIDS, have a rather short one. Such arguments constitute the logic underlying and motivating the Johns Hopkins Biographies of Disease.

But one must be cautious in deploying this metaphor. "Biography" implies a unified identity, a chronology, and a narrative— the movement of an entity in and through time. Biography implies visibility as well as unity and identity and thus recognition by contemporaries, and many ailments that we recognize in the twenty-first century do not fit easily into this implied narrative. This is particularly true in the case of ills whose manifestations are emotional and behavioral.

Allan V. Horwitz's study of what we have come to call PTSD and—mostly—accept as a coherent entity provides a particularly apt example of such an elusive story. Have we always had "PTSD" with us? In one sense yes, in another no. It is likely that men and women have always contended with the aftereffects of life-challenging, emotion-generating circumstances. Warriors in the world of classical antiquity could show signs of emotional problems after combat, but these were understood as issues of individual character, honor, and experience, not illness. In America's Civil War, Union and Confederate soldiers also showed signs of their particular war's impact. At least some of their symptoms, however, were framed as hypothetical physical pathology: "soldier's heart." In another mid-nineteenth-century context, the survivors of railroad accidents were understood as exhibiting the residual "nervous" effects of "spinal concussion." And, as is well known, the trench warfare of the First World War produced for a time an entity christened "shell-shock," another material and thus legitimate and morally exculpatory pathology. As is equally well-known, this term was soon seen as implausible because many soldiers showing postwar emotional signs had not been near the detonation of high explosives.

Throughout the period between the mid-nineteenth and early twentieth centuries, attitudes toward the survivors of trauma were beginning to be shaped not only by changing conceptions of disease in the medical profession but also by events in the public sphere: demands for soldiers' pensions in the case of veterans, or of the right of accident victims to take civil actions to seek compensation for their injuries in the case of railroad accidents. The extraordinary political mobilization created by the Vietnam War and its returning veterans provided another, late twentieth-century motivation for expanding notions of post-traumatic emotional pathology, putting flesh on the post-traumatic concept and activism behind its public articulation. Stress itself provided a mechanism, a black box of presumed physiological effects that promised the legitimacy of a material pathology underlying the emotional and behavioral symptoms that came to be lumped under the rubric of PTSD.

As Horwitz argues, the complex political process that supported a place for the diagnosis—and thus additional social visibility and plausibility for the disease concept—in the American Psychiatric Association's *Diagnostic and Statistical Manual of Mental Disorders* popularized the idea in the general population. PTSD remains in some ways contested, but it enjoys an increasingly well-recognized existence as a social as well as a pathological entity. With our past generation's increasing focus on non-war-related trauma—and especially sexual trauma—the PTSD concept has become an increasingly effective actor in the public sphere in today's battles over gender, as well as civil liability and government pension obligations. PTSD has an accepted place in today's cultural landscape, in the vocabulary of both policy debate and medical diagnosis. It is a social entity that can claim a biographical past—and a future.

Charles E. Rosenberg

When I entered graduate school to study psychiatric sociology in 1970, psychiatrists and sociologists shared an understanding that mental illness was grounded in social processes. At the time, both fields agreed that social influences were highly significant determinants of how mental disorder was defined, who became mentally ill, and the most effective ways to treat people with mental illnesses. Moreover, the role of biological factors in defining and explaining mental illness was virtually invisible, not just in sociology, but also in psychiatry. Like most sociologists, I celebrated the purely environmental post-traumatic stress disorder (PTSD) diagnosis that emerged in the third edition of the *Diagnostic and Statistical Manual of Mental Disorders* (*DSM-III*), in 1980. Unlike the other entities in this manual, which maintained a rigidly agnostic stance toward causation, the PTSD criteria assumed that social shocks could lead anyone—regardless of preexisting psychological or biological vulnerabilities—to become mentally disordered. The PTSD diagnosis seemed to vindicate the sociological project of framing mental illnesses within their sociocultural contexts.

From the vantage point of nearly half a century later, the prior dominance of social approaches seems thoroughly anomalous. Reductionist frameworks that find the essence of mental illnesses in brain regions, neurochemicals, and genes are ascendant in current research, treatment, and popular culture. PTSD, too, has been transformed from a condition rooted in social traumas to one grounded in the presumed brain changes it involves. In retrospect, it seems clear that the "brainless" psychiatry of the earlier period was just as intellectually shallow as is the "mindless" psychiatry of the current era. Both sociocultural and biological factors, as well as their interrelations, are critical aspects of all mental disorders.

This book uses the history of post-traumatic stress disorder to illustrate how the recent vicissitudes of definitions, explanations, and responses to mental illnesses reproduce conflicts that have continually marked the study of stressor-related conditions. PTSD provides an unusually clear lens that reveals the perennial alterations in psychiatric history between frameworks featuring, on the one hand, external exposure to stressors, sociocultural explanations, and environmental influences, or, on the other hand, individual vulnerabilities, biological mechanisms, and brain-based or psychologically based treatments. Likewise, it shows the recurrent conflicts between observers who have emphasized the reality of suffering that emerges from external shocks and others who have viewed stressor-based conditions as providing opportunities to evade responsibilities, displace blame, and reap compensation. No other psychiatric condition shows as clearly as PTSD does the competing frameworks that have been used to explore the nature of mental illness since the inception of psychiatry in the mid-nineteenth century.

A short history of a broad topic must be highly selective in the issues it features. I highlight three general themes: the problems that a stressor-related diagnosis poses for psychiatry and other mental health professions; the positive as well as the negative aspects of mental illness labels for their recipients; and the relative impact of biological and evaluative factors in definitions, explanations, and responses to mental illness. I focus on the central developments surrounding these issues regardless of where they occurred. This means that the book emphasizes European and British works at some points and American writings at others.

Fortunately, I have been able to draw on rich literatures in history, sociology, psychiatry, and psychology to explore the many fluctuations in views of PTSD and its predecessor diagnoses since their emergence a century and a half ago. I am particularly grateful to the following scholars for their insightful writings: Joan Acocella, Mikkel Borch-Jacobsen, Frederick Crews, Didier Fassin, Erin Finley, Christopher Frueh, Ian Hacking, Mardi Horowitz, John Kinder, Jerry Lembcke, Elizabeth Loftus, Kenneth MacLeish,

George Makari, Paul McHugh, Richard McNally, Mark Micale, David Morris, Richard Ofshe, Richard Rechtman, Gerald Rosen, Michael Roth, Sally Satel, Daniel Schacter, Wilbur Scott, Ben Shephard, Elaine Showalter, Michael Trimble, Jerome Wakefield, Simon Wessely, Alison Winter, and Allan Young. None, of course, is responsible for the uses to which I have put their work.

I have also greatly benefited from the assistance of a number of people connected with Johns Hopkins University Press. My initial editor, Jacqueline Wehmueller, helped to formulate the central thrust of the book and to sharpen the arguments of the completed manuscript. My current editor, Matt McAdam, helped to smoothly guide the book to publication. I am particularly indebted to Charles Rosenberg, the editor of the series of biographies of diseases in which this book appears, for his advice, from the book's initial conception through its final drafts. I am also grateful to the anonymous reviewers of the manuscript, who provided many helpful suggestions. Finally, Barbara Lamb has been an exceptionally able copy editor. All authors should be as lucky as I have been to work with such a supportive and skilled group of professionals.

PTSD

CHAPTER ONE

A Disorder through Time

At the beginning of the twenty-first century PTSD is
perhaps the fastest growing and most influential
diagnosis in American psychiatry.

Paul Lerner and Mark S. Micale, *Traumatic Pasts*

It is rare to find a psychiatric diagnosis that anyone likes
to have, but PTSD seems to be one of them.

Nancy Andreasen, "Posttraumatic Stress Disorder"

Post-traumatic stress disorder is the emblematic mental illness
of the early twenty-first century. PTSD marks the current era as
much as anxiety dominated the post–World War II period and
depression the two decades after the third edition of the *Diagnostic
and Statistical Manual of Mental Disorders* (*DSM-III*) was developed in 1980.[1] Traumas and their psychological consequences are
stock-in-trade of daytime talk shows, popular movies, television
documentaries, and news programs. A large industry has developed that encompasses trauma specialists, grief counselors, lawyers, and claimants. Laypersons routinely use the term "PTSD"
to describe their reactions to stressful events. For example, after

Donald Trump became president in 2016, one prominent writer asserted, "I swear I have developed P.T.S.D. from the venom of this election." Many mental health therapists reported a surge of traumatic cases after this election.[2]

As recently as 1980, the sorts of event that were considered to be "traumas" were limited to extreme stressors such as military combat, rape, severe assault, and natural or man-made disasters.[3] Since that time, the range of traumas has expanded to include hearing hate speech, learning of a relative's death, or watching a catastrophe unfold on television. Virtually the entire population experiences such "traumas" during their lifetimes. The number of individuals who develop PTSD after these events has also soared. In contrast to the initial studies of how many people suffer from PTSD, which showed rates of only about 1 percent, more recent reports indicate figures approximately ten times that number.[4]

Western and, increasingly, most cultures now routinely assume that people who are exposed to traumas will develop serious and recurrent negative psychological consequences. Mental health specialists typically predict that a pandemic of traumatic psychic conditions will arise after man-made and natural disasters.[5] As a result, trauma counselors have become entrenched in schools, work organizations, hospitals, and police and fire departments to deal with the expected psychological results of disturbing experiences. At the extreme, some instructors in colleges and universities use "trigger warnings" on reading material they feel might precipitate PTSD among their students.

The culture of PTSD has even penetrated the military, which long resisted the acceptance of stress-related conditions. During the mid-1990s and through the following decades, rates of treated PTSD among veterans rose to unprecedented levels. Between 2000 and 2013 the number of claimants in the Veterans Administration system receiving benefits for PTSD rose by almost 500 percent.[6] Compensation-seeking for this condition among veterans of the Iraq and Afghanistan Wars is orders of magnitude greater than among veterans of previous wars.[7] As a result of all these trends, according to historians Paul Lerner and Mark Micale, "at the beginning of the twenty-first century PTSD is perhaps the fastest growing and most influential diagnosis in American psychiatry."[8]

PTSD has become so embedded in current culture and medicine that it is easy to forget that the idea that traumas can cause mental disorders is a relatively recent notion. In contrast to depression, mania, and other conditions that have been recurrent medical and psychiatric concerns, PTSD and its predecessor diagnoses—soldier's heart, railroad spine, shell shock, and combat neurosis—only became recognizable psychiatric disorders in the latter part of the nineteenth century. Even then, claims of psychological trauma were commonly subject to suspicion and efforts to discredit them. The present expectation that dire and enduring psychological consequences will develop after stressful events stands in stark opposition to the resistance that traumatic diagnoses faced from both the medical establishment and the general culture for most of their brief history.

The relative newness of traumatic diagnoses contrasts with the perpetual presence of the kinds of event that produce PTSD. Combat, rape, severe physical assaults, disasters, serious accidents, and the like have been consistent occurrences throughout history. Indeed, violent conflicts, early deaths, sexual abuse, and disastrous natural calamities were far more common in past centuries than at present.[9] This raises the question of why PTSD has been considered to be a widespread medical problem only in recent periods.

Perhaps more than any other diagnostic category, PTSD is a vehicle for showing major historical changes in conceptions of mental illness. The inherent link between PTSD symptoms and traumatic events roots this condition in social and cultural forces to an unusually great extent among mental illnesses. Huge variations have existed over time about which conditions are likely to produce traumas, what are the results of traumas, who is susceptible to becoming traumatized, and how to evaluate the claims of trauma victims. The current Age of Post-Traumatic Stress Disorder is a product of changing views of the relationship of individuals to their environments and consequent notions of victimhood and vulnerability. The transformation of PTSD from a suspect to a ubiquitous psychiatric condition stemmed from reorientations in professional, cultural, and moral ideas about what constitutes a legitimate mental illness, what kinds of people can develop traumas, and what responses are appropriate for them. What, then, is PTSD?

DEFINING POST-TRAUMATIC STRESS DISORDER

Post-traumatic stress disorders have four central components. The first is that some external trauma has overwhelmed a person's capacity to cope with the experience. The term "trauma" itself stems from the Greek word for "wound," which connotes some injury or shock. In contrast to many mental illnesses that arise from some inner vulnerability, PTSD definitionally stems from a disturbance that is outside of the individual. Some traumas involve human agency, for example, combat, assaults, rapes, serious accidents, or terrorism; others stem from such natural causes as floods, hurricanes, or earthquakes. PTSD indicates a link between a prior negatively valued disruption and some present form of psychic suffering.

Because PTSD intrinsically entails some environmental trauma does not mean that individual and cultural interpretations of what is "traumatic" are irrelevant. Different people have highly variable thresholds of what they perceive as horrific or upsetting, so the emergence, nature, and severity of the traumatic event itself do not fully correspond to the intensity and persistence of post-traumatic symptoms. Personal appraisals of the traumatic quality of events themselves are heavily dependent on collectively held interpretations. Sharp boundaries between traumatic and nontraumatic stressors do not exist in nature. Different cultures draw lines in different places between events that expectably lead to pathological symptoms and those that do not; events that are traumatic in one place or time might be habitual in others. For example, battle was less of a shock in periods when violence was a routine part of life than in most modern Western societies, in which "a deep antipathy to violence and to conflict" exists.[10]

The second aspect of PTSD, its *post* quality, regards the temporal connection between recollections of some prior event, whether in the recent or the distant past, and some later psychological effect. Historically, there have been two major, sharply divergent ways of connecting traumas to their remembered psychic impacts. In the first conception, memories of past traumas recur in current experience with particularly powerful vividness, emotional charge, and repetitive quality. Anthropologist Allan Young observes that "time runs in the wrong direction, that is, from the present back to the past."[11] Sights and sounds activate recollections of earlier traumas with disturbing intensity, so people not only remember the trauma but actually relive it: "The event is happening *now*, in the *present*, for the *first time*."[12] Moreover, the past intrudes into the present in ways that are impossible for the person to control. Despite their efforts to push the traumatic event from consciousness, sufferers cannot escape its intrusive images. The force of such recollections leads people to become disconnected from their selves, from others, and from feelings of presence in their current lives.[13] In this view, traumatic experiences have such powerful impacts that they are difficult to forget.

In the second perspective, severely traumatic shocks can be so disturbing that victims are unable to remember them. This notion, which initially emerged in mid-nineteenth French psychiatry, has periodically reappeared to characterize the nature of traumatic memories. One prominent modern psychiatrist, Judith Herman, claims that "the ordinary response to atrocities is to banish them from consciousness."[14] Sufferers dissociate or repress their traumatic memories into a hidden part of the mind or brain, where they are still present yet are inaccessible to conscious recall. Sufferers and their therapists must make extensive and prolonged efforts, usually aided by some combination of hypnosis, drugs, and psychotherapy, to recover forgotten memories of the trauma. When this process is successful, recovered memories are recalled with perfect accuracy: "It is as though it comes from a photograph," Sigmund Freud proclaimed about such recollections.[15]

What unites these seemingly opposite notions is that memories of some past traumatic event, whether conscious or unconscious, lie behind the symptoms of PTSD.

The third component of PTSD, *stress*, involves the consequences that stem from experiences or recollections of traumatic events.[16] Some conceptions of stress focus on the particular psychic symptoms that define PTSD; others examine a much broader array of emotional, social, and behavioral impairments. The dominant current view, which is inscribed in the criteria of the *Diagnostic and Statistical Manual*, views PTSD as a specific memory-related disorder.[17] It ties stressful symptoms—including intrusive memories and disturbing dreams about the traumatic event, feeling upset about reminders of the event, unpleasant somatic sensations and heightened arousal when reexperiencing the trauma, and attempts to avoid recollections of traumatic circumstances—to the person's active memory of the traumatic event.

More generalized definitions of stressor-related disorders emphasize how external traumas typically lead to a range of damages that are not limited to memory-related conditions. Disrupted memory is just one feature of PTSD, and not necessarily even its central feature. Instead, traumatic events create more general social, psychic, and bodily difficulties. For example, psychiatrist Paul McHugh contends that PTSD is not a unique state but is instead an instance of a broader category of "emotions of adjustment," which also includes grief and homesickness, among others.[18] Adjustment implies that present problems comprise not just specific symptoms, such as vivid mental imagery, nightmares, and attempts to avoid recollections of the trauma, but also broader problems of social reintegration that involve reconciling recent and past circumstances. In this view, the temporal readjustments connected with PTSD usually naturally remit with the passage of time and changing circumstances. Optimal responses to problems of reintegration do not so much focus on dealing with memories of the past traumatic event as on providing supportive management of present troubles. "It is clear that the readjustment of the psychoneurotic is fully as much a social as a medical problem," sociologist Willard Waller wrote in 1944.[19]

Generalized definitions also emphasize how it is often very difficult to disentangle the symptoms of PTSD from those of other mental disorders, particularly anxiety and depression, because overwhelming majorities, often exceeding 80 percent, of people who have PTSD also meet criteria for other mental disorders.[20] PTSD can also be associated with behavioral expressions that include anger, violence, heavy drinking, and drug taking.

During the hundred years before the PTSD diagnostic criteria appeared in the *DSM-III* in 1980, psychiatrists usually viewed the symptoms of this condition as highly varied and heterogeneous. They included a diverse range of hysterical, anxious, and depressive states. Psychiatric definitions of PTSD subsequent to the *DSM-III* are far more specific and related to recurrent recollections of the trauma, avoidance of reminders of the trauma, and heightened arousal when remembering the trauma. While this notion of PTSD guides current research and treatment, the more general view that marked the previous hundred years is still influential. For example, the US government's Substance Abuse and Mental Health Services Administration, the federal agency charged with preventing and treating mental illness and substance abuse, still uses an extremely broad definition of trauma-related disorders: "Individual trauma results from an event, series of events, or set of circumstances that is experienced by an individual as physically or emotionally harmful or threatening and that has lasting adverse effects on the individual's functioning and physical, social, emotional, or spiritual well-being."[21] Likewise, recent lay conceptions are more likely to reflect an expansive view of the nature of PTSD than the particular memory-related definition found in the *DSM*.

Finally, *disorder* assumes that the symptoms resulting from traumatic exposure are pathological, not natural. Therefore, traumatic psychic consequences are framed within medical discourse as opposed to, say, defective character, sin, or some other form of moral interpretation. A medical definition implies that sufferers are not responsible for their distress and should be entitled to receive treatment and other resources.[22]

What distinguishes normal from disordered responses to traumas is often difficult to discern. Many observers have noted how the powerful human capacity for remembering trauma can be a naturally selected way of avoiding future dangers.[23] Experiences of periods of emotional numbness, vigilance, startle reactions, sleep difficulties, nightmares, intrusive images, and an avoidance of reminders associated with the trauma could reflect the inherent bias of fear mechanisms to reinforce and recollect rather than to forget past traumatic experiences. These extremely unpleasant responses can be normal reactions to insure that people remain alert to the possible recurrence of danger. For most people, such memories weaken over time, and disturbing symptoms slowly go away, although they might occasionally recur. Traumatic memories that do not diminish in intensity with passing years can indicate a disordered condition.

Each of the four elements of post-traumatic stress disorder raises central issues about how definitions of, explanations for, and responses to traumas have changed over time. They also generate key questions about the kinds of factor that produce mental disturbances, the moral judgments that are applied to mental illnesses, and the relationship of mental disorders to biology and culture.

PTSD: ENVIRONMENTAL STRESSORS OR INDIVIDUAL VULNERABILITIES?

Traumatic conditions have always been problematic diagnoses for psychiatry.[24] While psychiatric explanations have periodically emphasized how a heterogeneous range of social, moral, and lifestyle factors influence who becomes mentally ill, they generally regarded these environmental forces as precipitants of mental disorder in susceptible people. Early psychiatric thought was firmly rooted in hereditarian ideas: the causes of mental disorders were seen as originating from within individuals, usually those with an inherited predisposition to develop mental illness. Consequently, when the initial conceptions of traumatic neuroses began to emerge, mental disorders were viewed as diseases of the brain and nervous system.[25]

Stress-related diagnoses are distinct from psychiatry's traditional focus because they consider some external event as a necessary and, sometimes, sufficient cause of disorder. Traumatic conditions result from some shock outside of the afflicted person. Anyone who experiences traumatic events can be vulnerable to their effects, not just those who have some preexisting susceptibility. Post-traumatic stress disorder and associated conditions thus direct attention to how traumatic events themselves can cause mental disorder, challenging the profession's assumption that some inner weakness underlies pathology. Intense controversy traditionally surrounded the extent to which PTSD and its historical antecedents resulted from exposure to external disturbances or from internal vulnerabilities to stressors.

In contrast to exposure to external shocks, vulnerability implies that some earlier psychological state accounts for the consequences of traumatic experiences. Individual responses to even severe traumas have always varied widely; typically, only a minority, often a small minority, of people who are exposed to highly stressful circumstances display symptoms of PTSD. Others develop PTSD after only minor stressors. From the time when external traumas were first associated with lasting cases of mental illnesses, some observers regarded stressors as the primary causes of resulting symptoms while others viewed them as triggers of prior biological or psychological susceptibilities. This debate has been especially contentious during and after wartime: differing answers to the question of whether psychic injuries result from combat experiences or from aggravations of preexisting conditions are highly consequential for distinguishing truly deserving victims from those who have weak constitutions.

The environmental emphasis of stress-related diagnoses does not just challenge the psychiatric profession's typical ways of explaining mental disorder; it also calls into question the profession's therapeutic focus on changing vulnerable individuals as opposed to altering their social circumstances. Perhaps because of its environmental features, PTSD has always been one of the disorders most resistant to the therapeutic armamentarium of psychiatry. Psychoanalysts, for example, often shied away from treating victims of recent traumas.[26] Psychiatrists during World War I and World War II rarely used traditional therapies but instead provided brief periods of support and reassurance accompanied by adequate food, rest, and sleep to deal with post-traumatic symptoms.[27] Since the earliest recognition of traumatic conditions, drug treatments have periodically gained prominence, but none has proven to be very effective. The recalcitrance of PTSD to standard therapies continues into the present; current evaluations show that most psychotherapeutic and pharmacological techniques are unsuccessful.[28]

For much of its history, responses to PTSD focused on broader patterns of social reintegration rather than individual-oriented therapies. Especially when cases of PTSD stem from collective traumas, like wars and natural disasters, social and cultural factors shape reactions to an unusually great extent among mental disorders. Variables, including the strength of social networks of family and friends, the degree of available social support, the adequacy of economic circumstances, and the extent of current life difficulties, powerfully impact how trauma victims fare.[29] This is especially true for veterans who have fought in wars far away from their homes, often on different continents, making major problems of social readjustment inevitable. The environmental aspects of PTSD have often created difficulties in fully assimilating it into the psychiatric canon.

PTSD DIAGNOSES: STIGMATIZED OR VALUED?

The history of post-traumatic stress disorder has been inseparable from social movements and interest groups that both advocate and resist this diagnosis. On the one hand, it can be one of the few psychiatric diagnoses that is valued rather than stigmatized: "It is rare to find a psychiatric diagnosis that anyone likes to have, but PTSD seems to be one of them," psychiatrist Nancy Andreasen observes.[30] On the other hand, the same qualities that can make traumatic diagnoses highly valued in some situations also render them subject to suspicion precisely because of the rewards they can engender. The moral aspects of PTSD diagnoses tie them to cultural, social, and partisan considerations to an unusual extent among mental illnesses.

Examining the historical evolution of PTSD provides an especially good way of showing how valuations of psychiatric diagnoses sharply change in different historical periods. Diagnoses of mental illness have typically been associated with negative consequences—stigma, fear, shame, guilt. In contrast, the roots of PTSD in some external source can potentially cast blame and responsibility on some outer entity and so diminish the sufferer's own accountability. In particular, the intrinsic link of PTSD with some outside event brings issues of responsibility, blame, liability, and secondary gains into particularly sharp focus.

The emergence of psychological trauma as a psychiatric diagnosis called "railway spine" during the 1860s and 1870s was connected to the spread of mechanized technologies and to the resulting changes in conceptions of the obligation to redress harm when the malfunctioning of these technologies caused psychic injuries.[31] Although accidents have always led to much damage, insurance coverage for them only developed during the nineteenth century. Most importantly, railroads and the companies that insured them could be held liable for injuries resulting from the shock and trauma caused by train crashes.

Many sufferers of train accidents came to demand monetary compensation when their psychic conditions rendered them unable to resume their normal social roles. Skeptics challenged their claims and suggested that plaintiffs feigned their self-reported and unverifiable symptoms as ways to reap rewards and avoid responsibilities. For them, stressor-related diagnoses were associated with benefits that created powerful incentives to develop and maintain disabled states. The adversarial framework within which the initial traumatic complaints emerged shaped debates about these conditions for decades. Mental health professionals in the military, too, have always faced the dilemma that PTSD diagnoses provide excuses for soldiers to escape combat and the resulting possibility of death or serious injury. They can also lead to secondary gains, including pensions for as long as symptoms persist. Unsurprisingly, military institutions traditionally resisted the legitimacy of PTSD labels.[32]

Beginning in the 1960s, the post-traumatic stress disorder diagnosis became part of moral and legal crusades that involved sufferers' demands for redress. It was integrally connected to groups that questioned the wisdom of military involvements or, during the 1980s, challenged a culture of male sexual exploitation. Traumatized people, including soldiers, came to be seen as victims in need of help and deserving of assistance; people who questioned their suffering were seen as uncaring or immoral. The association of PTSD with broader political agendas firmly roots it in political conflicts as well as individual minds. It was difficult for medical personnel to remain neutral in these controversies, which are often related to secondary gains from the diagnosis of a disease and its accompanying sick role.[33]

The value placed on PTSD diagnoses has often sharply split along gendered lines. Gender differentiates many common traumas: combat provides the archetype for men, sexual assault for women. The history of moral evaluations of PTSD provides a particularly strong marker of dramatically changing views of masculinity. For millennia male responses to trauma, especially combat-related trauma, were foundational for conceptions of manhood. Cultural norms idealized men who acted courageously in potentially traumatic circumstances and harshly stigmatized those who responded in cowardly ways. Likewise, men were supposed "to keep quiet, forget the past, and move forward with their lives" after they experienced some trauma.[34] Until recently, traumatized men faced especially negative consequences when they received diagnoses of mental illnesses, including PTSD. In contrast, women have usually been far more receptive to interpreting their problems as signs of mental illness and to entering professional therapies. The association of patient roles with femininity and dependency was traditionally a source of social stigma and resistance to psychiatric treatment among traumatized males.[35]

Recently, the internalized cultural values that prevented men from overtly succumbing to trauma have started to break down, replaced by notions of victimization that previous notions of masculinity could not have incorporated. Newer ideas of manhood, which emphasize emotional connection and open expression of feelings, have largely supplanted older conceptions, which involve physical courage and stoicism. In particular, the idea that men who are psychologically damaged in combat must be cowardly has sharply altered to one in which men are viewed as victims deserving of sympathy and respect.[36] Traumatized men and women alike are easily assimilated into current therapeutic values, which emphasize weakness, expressiveness, and victimhood.

PTSD: GROUNDED IN BIOLOGY OR INTERPRETATIONS?

The historical study of post-traumatic stress disorder also provides a good lens through which to view fluctuations in the importance placed on biological or interpretative factors in definitions, explanations, and responses to mental illness. Stressor-related mental disorders bring to the fore the question of how much brains or minds account for the lingering effects of external traumas. Ever since the initial discussions over the nature of the psychic effects of train crashes, whether PTSD is based in biology or evaluative processes has been the source of intense disputes.

When psychiatrists began to consider the possibility that external traumas could produce severe psychological consequences, the field was firmly rooted in organic perspectives. Legitimate mental illnesses were associated with defective brains. The major problem that the initial students of stressor-related psychic disturbances confronted was how to tie the damage from severe external shocks, such as train crashes or exploding shells, to resulting psychological complaints. Then, as now, some observers focused on how powerful external stressors create neurological changes that in turn result in psychic symptoms. Indeed, the original terms for PTSD-type disorders, "railway spine" and "shell-shock," made explicit connections between an external trauma and an organic result.

Early neurologists were unable to find a neural signature of stressors. Their failure raised the issue of whether some purely mental process accounted for the endurance of symptoms after some outside shock. Students of trauma Jean-Martin Charcot and Pierre Janet posited that psychic rather than organic connections linked initial physical shocks with subsequent traumatic memories. They sought to uncover the unconscious memories of traumas they believed were responsible for the emergence and persistence of symptoms of hysteria much later in patients' lives. The debate over whether traumatic damage was physical or psychical persisted through World War I, with one side arguing that exploding shells led to real, albeit unobservable, changes in brains and the other that purely psychological states produced post-traumatic symptoms.

The issue of whether brains or minds connect external shocks to traumatic memories remains salient. The recent rise of neuroscience to a preeminent position in psychiatry and psychology has bolstered the position that PTSD is organically grounded. Neuroscientists strive to ground various types of distressing memories in particular brain locations, for example, the hippocampus and the amygdala.[37] Many, relying on brain-imaging technologies, assert that traumatic shocks lead to measurable biochemical and physiological effects on brain cells.

One implication of neuroscientific findings could be that PTSD must have existed long before it was explicitly recognized as a mental disorder. Because modern and ancient brains are virtually identical, the discovery of neural correlates of PTSD would indicate that it must have been present throughout history, well before it entered psychiatric nosologies in the late nineteenth century.[38] Using this line of reasoning, psychologists Yulia Ustinova and Etzel Cardeña assert that "the consistency of psychiatric reactions to combat stress throughout history is remarkable."[39] PTSD thus provides a lens to examine whether or not uncovering the neurobiological correlates of a mental disorder demonstrates that it has a timeless essence.

In contrast to the view that PTSD reflects neurological phenomena, many historians and social scientists emphasize how brains are not interchangeable with minds.[40] In this regard, the philosopher Ian Hacking has proposed an influential distinction, which is especially useful for the understanding of PTSD, between physical and cultural phenomena.[41] Varying descriptions of molecules, neurochemicals, or physiological forces do not change the ways that these things behave. Humans, however, respond dynamically to the concepts that define and interpret their actions. Therefore, their reactions to traumatic events are not independent of the frameworks they use to understand and explain them. A diagnosis of PTSD provides a model that traumatized people apply to shape what sort of experiences they have suffered, what kind of memories they should hold about them, and what type of responses they ought to make toward them. People in cultures that do not have diagnoses comparable to PTSD would not have unrecognized disease conditions but, instead, would experience traumas in entirely different ways. Thus, disease models do not just reflect but also actively shape the conditions that patients develop in any particular era.

Hacking's distinction implies that brains and minds are not identical: the same brain sensations would have profoundly different meanings and consequences among different individuals and across different cultures. Current neuroimaging technologies might uncover the brain locations where memories of traumatic events reside, but they cannot tell us anything about the content of these memories, what it feels like to experience them, or how they are expressed. Because equivalent neurological states can be associated with thoroughly different perceptions, feelings, and understandings, there would be little reason to think that the brain-based aspects of traumas lead to comparable conditions, especially across widely differing historical eras. Instead, appropriate explanations of past responses to trauma require knowledge of how people in earlier eras viewed them from their standpoint, not from ours.[42] "One of the difficulties in writing history," psychiatrist and historian Henri Ellenberger noted, "is that we are always prone to describe past events in terms of the meaning they have acquired in our time. But men of the past viewed contemporary events in their own perspective."[43]

To the extent that interpretations are important aspects of traumatic experiences, what is considered to be "traumatic" would differ widely across cultures. Events that are deeply disturbing in some cultures have no impact in others: falling into water is a trauma among the Bushmen of southern Africa, but not in Polynesia, where every child can swim.[44] Philosopher Mikkel Borch-Jacobsen provides the example of the Quechua Indians of Peru, who commonly develop symptoms of *Susto*, which strongly resemble those of PTSD, after becoming frightened by stimuli including thunder, the sight of a bull or snake, or sightings of old Incan ruins.[45] Such shocks, which are traumatic for the Quechua, would not be culturally appropriate reasons for developing PTSD symptoms among Westerners. Conversely, Borch-Jacobsen reports, a Quechua wouldn't develop symptoms of *Susto* after exposure to natural disasters or accidents that can provoke PTSD among Westerners.

From the interpretative viewpoint, current conceptions of PTSD deal with a condition in a way that simply was not available to people before the late nineteenth century. Anthropologist Allan Young contends that a new concept of a traumatic memory arose at this time, when it was "glued together by the practices, technologies, and narratives with which it is diagnosed, studied, treated, and represented and by the various interests, institutions, and moral arguments that mobilized these efforts and resources."[46] Such social practices and interpretations, not its location in the brain, are the primary forces accounting for the emergence of PTSD as a recognizable mental illness. The historical study of PTSD can help shed light on the extent to which traumas and their resulting symptoms are grounded in shocks that are based in biology, in interpretative processes, or in some combination of the two.

A DISORDER THROUGH TIME

The inherent link between external traumas and resulting symptoms inevitably leads PTSD to be inseparable from historical forces and social circumstances as well as from individual vulnerabilities. Each of the following chapters explores these connections through time.

Chapter 2 examines the emergence of the precursors of modern views of PTSD in the last decades of the nineteenth century. The first embryonic conceptions of battle trauma arose during the American Civil War, when extant cultural and medical norms had no framework for viewing this condition as a mental disorder. Nevertheless, instances resembling current cases of PTSD became plainly visible at the time. Train accidents provided a second, if highly controversial, source of the connection between external shocks and resulting psychic distress. "Railway spine" became the first medical diagnosis that associated traumas with subsequent psychological disturbances. Finally, within nineteenth-century medicine, traumas became well-known sources of mental problems in the work of Jean-Martin Charcot, Pierre Janet, and Sigmund Freud, which focused on women who experienced early, but repressed, traumas that led to psychic disturbances many years later.

The following chapter shows how World War I and World War II shaped conceptions of traumatic disorders for much of the twentieth century. These wars turned explanations of and treatments for traumas to contemporaneous disturbances rather than events that had occurred in the distant past. They also stimulated intense debates over the importance of exposure to environmental traumas as opposed to preexisting personal vulnerabilities in leading to psychic impairments. Finally, they moved the earlier focus on the traumatic ordeals of women to concentrate attention on the traumas of male combatants.

Chapter 4 highlights the drastic shift in social attitudes toward traumatic conditions during the post–World War II period through the 1970s. This change led to the purely event-based PTSD criteria that emerged in the *DSM-III* in 1980. The new diagnosis resulted from the lobbying efforts of Vietnam veterans and allied mental health professionals to insure that trauma victims were absolved from blame for their conditions and were able to secure therapy and disability payments. Although it has undergone substantial revisions since 1980, this diagnosis remains at the heart of current medical conceptions of PTSD.

The next chapter discusses the epidemic of traumatic diagnoses that developed among American women during the 1980s, which in many ways echoed the major concerns of late nineteenth-century European psychiatry. This decade marked the sudden emergence of a therapeutic corps devoted to recovering repressed memories of childhood sexual traumas among a clientele of suffering women. The focus of PTSD-related conditions sharply turned from male victims of combat to female victims of male abuse. The equally abrupt decline of the recovered memory movement during the 1990s illustrates the power of therapeutic suggestion in bringing about traumatic conditions.

The penultimate chapter explores the huge growth of PTSD since the 1990s. The rise of a therapeutic culture has greatly expanded the sorts of trauma that are assumed to cause PTSD, the number of people they afflict, and the conditions that warrant therapeutic responses. The result is that PTSD has become a signature mental disorder of our age.

The book concludes with an examination of how the history of PTSD can help illuminate a number of central issues about mental disturbances more generally. These include the relative importance of external stressors and internal vulnerabilities in generating mental illness, the benefits and costs of mental illness labels, and the interrelationships of biology and culture in shaping the nature of mental illness.

CHAPTER TWO

PTSD Emerges

Shell-shock had not yet been heard of, but families recognized
that after cannonade and bayonet charge a man might come
home and seem queer for a while. The warp of battle might
remain in him for a long time.

Dixon Wecter, *When Johnny Comes Marching Home*

A man, whose spine is concussed on a railway, brings an action
against the company, and does or does not get heavy damages. A
man, who falls from an apple-tree and concussed his spine, has—
worse luck for him—no railway to bring an action against.

British Medical Journal, December 1, 1866

Hysterics suffer mainly from reminiscences.

Sigmund Freud and Josef Breuer, *Three Studies in Hysteria*

Before the mid-nineteenth century no diagnosis resembling post-
traumatic stress disorder existed in the psychiatric canon. The psychic aftereffects of traumatic shocks would have been formulated
through some nonmedical discourse such as moral character or
religion, if at all. At the time, biological perspectives dominated

European and American psychiatry. German psychiatrist Wilhelm
Griesinger's (1817–69) dictum that "mental diseases are brain diseases" captured the essential assumption of the field. Neurologists, too, optimistically believed that they were on the threshold
of discovering the mysteries of mental disorder within the brain.
Franz Joseph Gall's (1758–1828) phrenology and Pierre Paul Broca's (1824–80) localization of memory in discrete sections of the
brain led researchers to seek the specific organic centers that corre-
sponded to different sorts of mental illness. Anticipating modern
neuroscience, they strove to reduce psychic life to the activity of
the brain and the nervous system. As long as mental phenomena
were firmly rooted in internal physiological processes, it was difficult for a psychiatric diagnosis grounded in external traumas to
emerge.

Several developments in the latter half of the century brought
to the fore a new conception of psychic damage that did not easily fit the existing reductionist framework. In particular, three
distinct factors led to the common, if controversial, recognition
that external shocks could lead to traumatic psychological consequences. First, the carnage of the American Civil War created
an embryonic, usually latent, conception that combat-related
traumas could produce lasting mental consequences. In addition,
widespread industrialization led to many accidents, especially railway crashes, which induced psychic shocks. Finally, the notion
that repressed memories of childhood traumas could produce hysterical symptoms in later life became a central tenet of European
psychiatry. By the turn of the century, traumas and their psychic
consequences were well-recognized not only within the psychiatric profession but also in the general culture. The controversies
that developed in this era about how to distinguish symptoms that
arose from traumas from those that resulted from preexisting vulnerabilities, from hopes for secondary gains, or from therapeutic
suggestion remain central to current discussions of PTSD.

THE AMERICAN CIVIL WAR

The American Civil War provided one turning point in the history of PTSD.[1] At the time, legitimate combat injuries were limited to physical wounds. No medical framework existed that could encompass emotional damage from warfare. Instead, conceptions of character provided the primary lens for evaluating psychic disability. Psychologically damaged men who were unable to fight were reviled as cowards. "Men pity them; women despise them," the *New York Times* editorialized in 1861.[2] They were seen as malingerers who dishonorably pretended to be sick in order to evade combat.

The first cracks in this characterological view, however small, appeared during and in the aftermath of this war. It was one of the first to utilize modern weaponry, including repeating rifles, heavy artillery, and high explosives. Hand-to-hand combat was also common. The war featured massive slaughter: there were nearly 23,000 casualties in a single day at Antietam; the three-day battle of Gettysburg generated 50,000 deaths. Bullets, often fired at close range, caused almost all (94 percent) combat wounds, and artillery shells were responsible for the remainder.[3] Overall, the Union and Confederate forces suffered more than 600,000 fatalities, equivalent to 6 million deaths today. On a proportionate basis, this was six times more than in World War II, thirty one times more than in the Korean War, and sixty-nine times more than in the Vietnam War.[4]

Most Civil War combatants had experienced little exposure to violence before they entered battle. Almost all were volunteers, not professionals. Most were very young, many teenagers, often just entering their teen years. Many also had to overcome internalized religious prohibitions against killing. The new technologies of warfare had unprecedented psychological consequences for such untested youths, who could not have been prepared for the mass slaughter that many witnessed. Soldiers also faced wretched physical conditions marked by high rates of disease—especially dysentery—vile living situations, and unpredictable food supplies. More men died from disease than from combat.[5]

During the Civil War itself, few soldiers were judged to be insane: of the roughly 2 million Union soldiers, only about 1,200 entered the federal mental hospital at St. Elizabeth's. Overall, official records indicated that less than 1 percent of soldiers suffered from nervous diseases, including not just insanity but also milder conditions, which were often called "nostalgia" or "sunstroke."[6] Few of even this small number of conditions were attributed to combat. "Nostalgia," a condition that featured loss of appetite, profound sadness, and constant longing for home, was regarded as the result of the loss of peacetime connections as opposed to the war itself. It was especially common among youth who had never been away from their families and who weren't mature enough to cope with war.[7] "Sunstroke" was another extremely broad diagnosis that might have been a synonym for what later came to be called "combat fatigue."[8] Neither of these conditions, however, had presentations that resemble current PTSD symptoms or any connection to memory disorders. Nor did they resonate with cultural conceptions regarding psychological outcomes of combat. "Diagnostic language undoubtedly aided veterans at a loss to give a name to their ailments, but ultimately had little influence with the public at large," historian Brian Jordan observes.[9]

Nor did the notion that soldiers could suffer from combat-related mental illness take root in military medicine. Both officers and physicians viewed psychiatric casualties as malingerers: "The letters, diaries, and memoirs of these medical men generally reflect almost a zeal to implement the official policy of detecting cases of feigned insanity in soldiers seeking to escape combat or to secure a discharge from the service."[10] Soldiers who refused to enter combat, regardless of their reasons, were subject to harsh punishments.

If the military disdained claims of mental distress, most soldiers and their families used the broader cultural framework of "masculinity, patriotism, and religion," and especially of sacrifice, to interpret their experiences: "I came into this war to lay down my life," explained one soldier.[11] The desire to avoid labels of cowardice was an especially intense motivation for shunning any expressions of psychological breakdown. Cowards faced intense disgrace and were regarded with contempt as "despicable shirkers."[12] Union general Francis Patterson provides one example. Patterson begged off sick before a battle and, faced with court martial, shot himself in 1862. In another case, the father of an officer who deserted his men wrote his son that he would be better off if he were dead.[13]

Despite the absence of any extant cultural or medical explanatory frameworks for a traumatic mental condition, there are indications that some soldiers developed PTSD-like symptoms. In one instance, Horace Porter, an aide to General Ulysses Grant, noted that after combat, soldiers "would start at the slightest sound, and dodge at the flight of a bird or a pebble tossed at them."[14] Hospital records also indicate scattered cases of postcombat mental disturbances. A nurse recorded an encounter with "an insane man" who struggled with "his battles over again." This veteran "fought the rebels all day, tearing his bed and clothes until exhausted."[15] The records of one veteran who was committed to an Indiana mental hospital noted that he was "restless and sleepless, suicidal. Attempted suicide. Imagines he is bleeding to death from imaginary wounds."[16] Another nurse at a Union hospital described a patient's nightmares, "as they all are, he was on the battlefield, struggling to get away from the enemy."[17] But such explicit references to bad dreams or disturbed sleep were rare.[18] Common assumptions at the time led personnel to interpret possibly psychic symptoms as manifestations of physical, not psychological, problems.[19] Because war-related psychopathology did not conform to any recognized diagnostic category, symptoms that would now be recognized as possible signs of PTSD appear only sporadically in hospital records.

Postwar Developments

Most veterans faced miserable conditions after the war had ended. Postwar life was especially abysmal in the defeated South, which featured a decimation of its male population, the general destruction of property, a ruined infrastructure, and widespread poverty. About a quarter of white Southern males were dead. The war had destroyed two-thirds of the value of Southern wealth. Conditions of near starvation and homelessness were common.[20] Information about psychic casualties among Confederate veterans is sparse— the postwar devastation was so pervasive that it overshadowed any concern with psychological issues among veterans.[21] In any case, Confederate veterans were ineligible for pensions or any other kind of compensation from the federal government and so had no motivation to report traumatic symptoms.[22]

In the North, too, postwar social conditions featured high unemployment and inflation. Many veterans were young, without property, and jobless. After the initial celebrations and parades were over, the notion that impaired veterans were nuisances dominated. Disabled bodies were stigmatized as "economically burdensome, psychologically unstable, and socially objectionable."[23] The primary concern of the public became the costs, diseases, and moral maladies that they associated with veterans.[24] Most doctors in the postwar period also considered psychological problems to be signs of personal and moral failure, cowardice, loss of character, or malingering rather than medical results of wartime experiences.[25]

Many veterans turned to alcohol, laudanum, or opiates to dull memories of the war's horrors. Alcoholism was the worst problem, the "veterans' most stubborn enemy."[26] Others, especially in Eastern cities, sought help from neurologists. In the absence of any particular diagnosis for traumatic psychic conditions, they were often given the nonspecific diagnosis of "nerves."[27] Beginning in the late 1860s many veterans, like civilians more generally, received the new, extraordinarily capacious diagnosis of "neurasthenia," which was related to preexisting constitutional predispositions, not to traumatic experiences.[28]

As some veterans' symptoms persisted with the passage of time, physicians continued to resist attributing postwar mental afflictions to prior combat involvements. Some connected symptoms to personal or moral failings.[29] Others employed diagnoses related to physical explanations. The heart garnered the most attention as the source of impairment.[30] Physician Jacob Da Costa

(1833–1900) was the most prominent observer of veterans' maladies. Da Costa famously coined the term "irritable heart" to refer to a syndrome featuring hyperventilation, heart palpitations, very high pulse rate, and shortness of breath that were not due to any recognizable organic disease. This label avoided any psychic tinge and was thus acceptable to patients and physicians alike. In line with prevailing medical theories at the time, Da Costa and other doctors didn't link the condition to postcombat stress but to either physical overexertion or predisposing factors, including family history, weak constitutions, or infections.[31]

Despite the obstacles to interpreting psychic symptoms as results of combat, the aftermath of the Civil War featured the first stirrings of psychological interpretations of wartime experiences. One notable aspect was that this was the first conflict in which a high proportion of soldiers were literate, so considerably more written material describes their personal combat and postwar experiences than was available in previous wars. Even if physicians and the public failed to recognize postwar psychic conditions, these letters show that veterans themselves and their immediate family members often did.

Many veterans wrote about how the intense strain of battle persisted over time, causing intrusive recollections, startle reactions, and nightmares. Some men relived traumatic events that were a "frequent and debilitating complaint that most civilians failed to understand."[32] A survivor of the carnage at Shiloh proclaimed: "Tho it now lacks but two days of forty two years since that morning, the picture has not faded in the least."[33] Another recalled that he relived the horror of combat, "every year of my life since (I have) borne it all with a mighty small amount of sympathy from those about me."[34] Several years after the war, the wife of a Union soldier recounted how her husband would cry out: "Don't speak to me; don't you hear them bombarding? . . . They are coming, they are coming. See the bombshell."[35] In 1881, well after the war had ended, another veteran of combat stated: "My flesh trembles, and creeps, and crawls when I think of it today. My heart almost ceases to beat at the horrid recollection."[36] Renowned

essayist Ambrose Bierce was "haunted all his life by what he described as persisting 'visions of the dead and dying.' "[37]

Civil War historians who have studied the psychic effects of
the war consistently note the scale of the problem. One claims
that, "haunted by their wartime experiences, countless veterans
endured paranoia, chronic depression, and debilitating flashbacks
for years afterward."[38] Another emphasizes that combat memories
were "something that [soldiers] lived with every day."[39] Historian
Michael Adams concludes: "Actually, every description of psychiatric wound identified since 1914 had precedent in the 1860s."[40]

Compensation

Obtaining compensation was the major hurdle facing veterans
with persistent and debilitating psychic symptoms. The most important controversy regarding Civil War veterans related to pensions. While veterans were viewed as heroic, courageous, and self-
sacrificing, they were also expected to quickly adjust to civilian
life without placing undue demands on the state or the public.
In the eyes of their communities, they should return home and
carry on with their lives as if nothing untoward had happened to
them.[41]

It was extraordinarily difficult for psychically damaged veterans to secure a pension. One reason was that mentally traumatized
veterans who had no visible signs of injury were disqualified.[42] Another was that government compensation was disallowed if appli-
cants had "immoral" habits, including alcohol and drug abuse or
masturbation.[43] Such traits were associated with character weaknesses, not with medical conditions. A third was that reception
of a pension required showing a direct connection between some
specific wartime event and some subsequent psychological trauma
and its continuance. The assumption that there must be a direct,
unbroken causal link to battle limited the ability to claim disability. If too long a lapse between the event and its consequences
existed, then the claim was discredited. For example, one pension
board ruled that a veteran's family was not entitled to compensation: "Rejection, on the ground that soldier's death from suicide

in 1875 can in no way be attributed to his military service from which he was discharged in 1865."[44] It is likely that most psychically impaired veterans who did receive pensions claimed them through coexisting physical problems and diseases that they suffered in the war rather than through their mental disturbances.[45] The anticipation of compensation for psychic disabilities did not shape Civil War veterans' reports of traumatic symptoms.

The view that it was unmanly for veterans to be dependent on the government also shaped official policies. In 1887 President Grover Cleveland vetoed a pension bill, stating that the vast majority of Union veterans had "contentedly resumed their places in the ordinary avocations of life" but that a small minority wanted to be "simple objects of charity."[46] Nevertheless, vigorous advocacy by veterans' organizations and supportive politicians led Benjamin Harrison, who succeeded Cleveland, to sign the pension bill into law in 1890, although many felt it would "stimulate dishonesty and dependency."[47] The enormous cost of the Civil War pension system was seen as a serious problem. In 1893, the United States was spending more than 40 percent of its total annual budget on benefits for nearly 1 million war pensioners. By the time the country entered World War I, in 1917, it had spent over $8 billion on pensions.[48] Although few pensioners made explicitly psychological claims, subsequent discussions of traumatic neuroses were framed within the context of the tremendous potential burden they would place on national budgets.

There is little doubt that many Civil War soldiers suffered serious psychological damage in and after combat. Yet, the medical profession, the culture at large, and most veterans themselves were not yet ready to assimilate mental illness to conceptions of appropriate soldierly conduct. No extant medical diagnosis could encompass the psychic aftershocks of battle. Moreover, the potential budgetary burden of psychically disabled soldiers stymied the common use of any PTSD-like diagnosis. Concern regarding the costs of pensions for mental afflictions reinforced the skepticism surrounding postcombat psychological conditions. Another development, however, was emerging in civil society that would help propel PTSD-related conditions to the attention of physicians and the general public.

RAILROADS

The Industrial Revolution and the associated development of motorized transportation provided a major impetus for the modern conception of traumatic psychological conditions. Before the nineteenth century, no corporate entity had either the social responsibility or legal liability for the damage they created. This situation dramatically changed with the mechanization connected with the new social order. While industrialization led to numerous accidents in factories, buildings, mines, and other work sites, railway accidents in particular captured public attention.[49] The vast increase in train traffic beginning in the 1840s led to many wrecks and resultant litigation against the large corporations that owned the railroads. As public concern with the rising number of injuries from train and other industrial accidents grew, medical conceptions of psychic trauma began to change.[50] By the 1870s physicians were actively debating the nature of traumas and their psychological consequences. The consequences of the Industrial Revolution forced medical professionals to reexamine their bedrock beliefs in the hereditary foundations of mental disturbances.

The central conflict that arose during this period was between doctors who believed that psychological symptoms emerging after accidents were products of organic damage, on the one hand, or were mental phenomena without a somatic basis, on the other. British surgeon John Erichsen's *On Railway and Other Injuries of the Nervous System* (1866) was the first medical text to explore this condition in detail. Erichsen (1818–96) believed that railway accidents were not unique but were an especially powerful and violent type of trauma.[51] He posited that crashes produced spinal compression, which in turn resulted in emotional symptoms. Erichsen understood the controversial nature of what he called "concussion of the spine": "There is indeed no class of cases in which medical men are now so frequently called upon to give evidence in the courts of law, as those which involve the many intricate questions that arise in actions for damages against railway companies for injuries of the nervous system, alleged to have been sustained by passengers in collisions; and there is no class of cases in which more discrepancy of surgical opinion may be elicited."[52] Erichsen testified on behalf of victims who sued railway companies for damages, emphasizing how post-traumatic conditions were grounded in somatic damage that was analogous to brain concussions. They featured a wide variety of symptoms, including rigid limbs, back pain, insomnia, confusion, and fatigue. While many of these symptoms closely resembled hysteria, this female-related diagnosis was inappropriate for the mainly male victims of train crashes. In addition, at the time hysteria was connected to biological predispositions, so crash victims would not receive compensation for conditions that were called "hysterical."[53] For this male clientele, a new diagnosis of "railway spine" was more congruent with conventional gender roles. In line with the prevailing organic model of mental disorder, Erichsen attributed the problems associated with this condition to the presence of lesions in the brain or spinal cord.[54]

Some commentators accepted the legitimacy of psychic symptoms, although others equated them with malingering. The latter group emphasized that people could easily fabricate psychological impairments that had no visible signs. There was no question about the objective nature of the loss of an arm, leg, or eye as a result of an accident; moreover, a precise sum could be placed on the damages due for such harms.[55] Yet, subjective reports of psychic impairments were unverifiable and subject to simulation. This feature led to intense criticism of Erichsen's belief in the reality of psychic damage. One skeptical reviewer of his book contended that "the only differences which . . . are to be found between railway and other injuries are purely incidental and relate to their legal aspects. A man, whose spine is concussed on a railway, brings an action against the company, and does or does not get heavy damages. A man, who falls from an apple-tree and concussed his spine, has—worse luck for him—no railway to bring an action against."[56] In this view, the distinctive aspect of railway psychic injuries was to provide opportunities for monetary reward.

Another line of attack against Erichsen stemmed from the position that psychic injuries resulting from train crashes arose through mental, not physical, mechanisms. In the United States, prominent neurologist James Jackson Putnam contended that the psychic aftereffects of train crashes were akin to the psychological condition of hysteria.[57]Another American physician noted: "More than the physical injury in these cases, there seems to be psychical effect, either immediately accompanying the accident, such as the horrible sight of suffering, the cries of the injured, the agony of the mangled bodies, and all sorts of horrible scenes; in addition to that, even if not injured himself, come the terror of personal danger, the mental agony, the fright, etc., affecting the victim profoundly."[58] In this vein, English surgeon Herbert Page argued against Erichsen that nervous shocks resulted from purely mental origins: "In these purely psychical causes lies, we believe, the explanation of the remarkable fact that after railway collisions the symptoms of general nervous shock are so common, and often so severe, in those who have received no bodily injury."[59] Only a few cases, Page argued, resulted from observable organic damage.

The emergence of psychic symptoms could be delayed: some people who were unscathed in the aftermath of a crash only became impaired well after the time of the accident. Novelist Charles Dickens, who experienced a train accident, wrote about its deferred consequences: "I am not quite right within, but believe it to be an effect of the railway shaking. There is no doubt of the fact that, after the Staplehurst experience, it tells more and more (railway shaking, that is) instead of, as one might have expected, less and less."[60]

The question that participants in this controversy tried to answer was, "How to understand a wound that refused to heal yet remained invisible?"[61] To what was the nervous system responding when it still produced symptoms after lengthy periods of time had passed since the accident had taken place? The idea developed that the missing link between the original trauma and long-standing psychic symptoms was not the original event itself but the patient's *memory* of it. Although not clearly formulated, this view was a predecessor of the modern notion that views PTSD as a disorder of memory.

During last third of the nineteenth century, the idea that sudden physical shocks could lead to purely mental problems and to psychologically based diseases began to take hold. According to historians Mark Micale and Paul Lerner, a "progressive mentalization of the trauma concept" occurred over the course of this period.[62] Emphasis shifted from physical to psychological factors as traumas came to be viewed not as external events per se but as the experiencing and remembering of the event in an individual's mind. Traumatic neuroses began to be consolidated as a distinct psychiatric category: "Psychological trauma acquired the status of a disease entity with a technical terminology, theories of causation, a classification, and therapeutic systems as well as medico-legal standing and governmental recognition."[63]

The new mental conception of trauma did not displace the deeply rooted somatic and hereditarian views that remained dominant in nineteenth-century medicine. In accord with existing hereditarian views, proponents of both the physical and psychic views of trauma accepted the importance of prior personality and degree of constitutional nervousness as predictors of which shock victims might develop traumatic neuroses. Indeed, historian Eric Caplan contends that, "rather than provide a psychological explanation for what were indisputably post-traumatic symptoms, the overwhelming majority of physicians offered instead a compelling materialistic explanation for the various symptoms their patients displayed."[64] By the end of the century, opinions were sharply split between those who adhered to Erichsen's position, that railway spine was grounded in some physical injury, and others, who adhered to psychologically oriented etiologies of the symptoms associated with this condition.

Liability

The notion of "railway spine" brought issues of liability to the fore. The debate regarding the nature of traumatic psychic conditions emerged in the context of litigation, responsibility, and accountability. Trains not only caused the traumas leading to symptoms, but railroad companies had insurers with pockets deep enough to provide compensation to accident victims. In 1870 one British physician noted: "Hitherto our experience has been derived almost wholly from litigated cases, deformed by contradictory statements and opinions; and the verdicts of juries have stood in the place of post-mortem reports."[65] Starkly competing frames emerged that emphasized either suffering victims who deserved compensation or malingerers who simulated symptoms to get monetary rewards.

The center of contention was whether those who claimed psychic injuries from train crashes were entitled to compensation. In 1879 German psychologist C. T. J. Rigler introduced the term "compensation neurosis" to explain the rise in disabled cases after train accidents.[66] While both malingerers and hysterics realized gains from symptoms, malingerers, but not hysterics, were conscious of their deceit.[67] A Boston surgeon, Richard Manning Hodges, argued that the persistence of trauma-related symptoms was due "not to the specific peculiarities of train accidents, but to the annoying litigation and exorbitant claims for pecuniary damage that are constantly the grave result of their existence."[68]

Physicians who testified in court had to prove a precise causal connection between an accident and resultant psychological symptoms among suffering complainants.[69] Yet, unlike physical disabilities, psychic wounds were not visible apart from patient reports. Typical legal cases featured plaintiffs' lawyers who emphasized the seriousness of psychic injuries and the depth of their client's suffering, and corporate defendants who associated psychological wounds with malingering. Each side called upon doctors who testified that injuries were either profound or nonexistent.[70] Victims' arguments generally proved to be more powerful than those of corporate defendants. By 1877 British juries had awarded over $11 million in damages to people who claimed that railway accidents had caused railway spine. In the United States, as well, hostility toward corporations led American juries to rule for plaintiffs in about 70 percent of cases.[71]

The initial battles over the reality of psychic traumas were thus mainly fought in courtrooms. The locus of contention in Europe changed with the emergence of workmen's compensation and pensions toward the end of the nineteenth and beginning of the twentieth century. In Great Britain, the 1911 National Insurance Act provided general compensation for sickness, regardless of liability issues. Once governments became responsible for reimbursing accident victims, these victims no longer needed to sue corporate defendants. In 1889 the German Insurance Officer recognized post-traumatic neuroses as compensable, and people with symptoms of traumatic hysteria, among others, began to make claims for pensions. The invisible nature of psychic traumas became a particular concern of those who feared a surge in disability claims for traumatic mental illnesses. Many observers believed that secondary gains from "pension neuroses" would lead injured people to exaggerate the severity and persistence of their symptoms to reap greater financial rewards.[72]

The next three decades witnessed "a bitter political fight over the veracity of pension neuroses," one that resembled the debate between Erichsen and his critics.[73] Berlin neurologist Hermann Oppenheim (1858–1919) was the best-known participant. He developed a theory of traumatic neurosis as a distinct diagnosis, the direct result of traumatic experience and not a hysterical or psychogenic reaction.[74] Like Erichsen, Oppenheim deemphasized subjects' ideas and thoughts and focused on organic shocks as causes of symptoms. Oppenheim's critics emphasized how a diagnosis of traumatic neurosis guaranteed a pension at the public's expense. They claimed that, regardless of the original cause of symptoms, the promise of material and psychic gains led the symptoms to endure. Some asserted that a mass epidemic of "pension addiction" occurred because workers were encouraged "to be as sick as possible." As one report noted, "without the existence of liability laws of any kind, accident or other avaricious pension neuroses would entirely not exist."[75] A consensus eventually formed against Oppenheim that the social insurance bureaucracy had led to a proliferation of exaggerated claims of psychoneuroses.[76]

By the end of the nineteenth century two distinct schools had developed. The first followed Erichsen in the view that traumatic psychic injuries were organically based and genuine. The other, echoing Page, saw them as psychological and often falsified. These contrasting positions shaped controversies about the nature of psychic traumas for many decades thereafter.

PSYCHIATRY

Developments in European psychiatry during the last half of the nineteenth century provided the third and, ultimately, most influential source of the current PTSD diagnosis. Although the grounding of the mind in the brain had dominated psychiatric thought since the 1700s, a nascent, more psychic conception of the mind was emerging. Viennese physician Moritz Benedikt (1835–1920) initially focused medical attention on the role of painful, usually sexual, repressed secrets that underlay many cases of hysteria.[77] The idea that people hid traumatic memories not only from others but also from themselves was new. This conception also raised the disturbing prospect that memories could have effects that were independent of consciousness.[78] Around the same time, French philosopher and psychologist Théodule-Armand Ribot (1839–1916) developed the idea that certain types of forgetfulness led to states of "double consciousness," which could have pathological consequences.[79]

Especially in France, memory disturbances became a prominent focus of scientific research, as well as a topic of broader cultural interest. French neurologists, psychiatrists, and psychologists came to focus on the disorders of hysteria, amnesia, and multiple personality, all of which involved problems with memory and people's relationships with their pasts. The idea that the mind contained a duality of conscious and unconscious psychological processes was beginning to enter the corpus of medical knowledge.[80]

During the last part of the nineteenth century, the idea of the unconscious and its accompanying theoretical and therapeutic implications became the cornerstone of a new dynamic psychiatry. The dynamic approach assumed that memories of past traumas were often at the root of present psychopathologies.[81] Debates focused on where the past was when we were not conscious of it. At the same time, hypnotic techniques were used to bridge the present and the past. This was the atmosphere in which French neurologist Jean-Martin Charcot developed his influential work on the neurological and psychological potency of what was not remembered.

Charcot

Neurologist Jean-Martin Charcot (1825–93) was the most prominent medical figure dealing with mental illness, hysteria in particular, during the period between 1878 and his death in 1893. Hysteria was a broad label that referred to a wide variety of psychic and physical symptoms, including paralysis, fainting, convulsions, seizures, choking, and emotional outbursts. One of Charcot's major contributions was to take a previously incoherent mass of symptoms and turn them into a clear diagnosis of hysteria. Charcot thus raised the profile of post-traumatic symptoms by associating them with hysteria, the "ur-neurosis of fin-de-siècle medicine."[82] He believed that some intense past trauma precipitated such symptoms, although he thought that external events were triggers of hysteria among people who were already biologically predisposed to develop this condition, rather than independent causes of it.

Charcot's thinking was embedded in nineteenth-century hereditarian conceptions of mental illness, which emphasized how only biologically vulnerable people were likely to develop hysteria. Charcot, however, departed from prevailing medical thought in resisting the common notion that gynecological problems caused hysteria, meaning that this condition was found only in women. Unlike most previous conceptions, Charcot insisted that, although hysterics were usually female, men as well as women could develop this condition. A number of Charcot's patients were men whose symptoms had emerged after some traumatic shock, often as employees or passengers involved in train wrecks: "These serious and obstinate nervous states which present themselves after (railway) collisions, and which render their victims incapable of working . . . are very often hysteria," he wrote.[83] Charcot's formulation, which encompassed men as well as women, allowed him to transfer the legitimate providers of care for hysterics from gynecologists to neurologists.

Charcot postulated that memories of past shocks were often not conscious but lingered in the unconscious, becoming manifest through hysterical symptoms. Although some of his patients suffered from traumas of child abuse and rape, Charcot did not focus on sexual traumas and rarely mentioned sexuality at all. Instead, he emphasized that the environmental precipitants provoking hysteria were marked by their unexpectedness, combined with hereditary predilections to defective nervous systems. This emphasis, however, varied by sex: predispositions were more important for women, while triggering events like train wrecks had greater importance for men.[84]

Charcot's celebrity resulted from his public demonstrations of the power of hypnotic treatments at a Parisian hospital, the Salpêtrière. He put his female hysterics on display in lectures during which they performed before large crowds. These events, which were the focus of intense cultural and medical attention, involved extravagant displays of hysterical fits by his female patients. In them, Charcot hypnotized his patients so that they would remember the repressed traumas that presumably lay behind their problems. Once forgotten memories had been uncovered in hypnotic sessions, he thought they would become open for use by normal processes of recollection. Although Charcot's showmanship made him one of the most prominent celebrities of his time, his particular ideas about heredity and trauma did not last. His major contribution was to legitimate the idea that traumas could trigger, although rarely cause, hysterical neuroses.

Railway spine raised the question of whether victims' claims resulted from genuine shocks or from malingering and desires for compensation. In contrast, the central controversy over Charcot's work was the extent to which medical suggestion led patients to display hysterical symptoms in order to please their clinicians. It was not difficult to feign indicators of hysteria. One of Charcot's students, Joseph Babinski, observed that patient presentations reflected those symptoms they thought Charcot wanted to see.[85] Indeed, his patients competed to exhibit the most vivid displays in order to get his attention.[86] The conventional portrait of the hysterical patient became a woman with "hair disheveled, head tossed back, limbs contorted, eyes rolling, and body rigid and writhing."[87] Babinski contended that once physicians stopped reinforcing such exhibitions they would disappear. A rival of Charcot's, Hippolyte Bernheim, accused Charcot of using hypnosis as a way of implanting memories of traumas that had never occurred rather than of eliciting real memories. The power of physicians to evoke iatrogenic traumatic symptoms would often recur in the history of PTSD.

Janet

Although French psychologist Pierre Janet (1859–1947) is currently viewed as a less influential progenitor of the post-traumatic stress disorder diagnosis than Charcot or Sigmund Freud, during the late nineteenth century his renown equaled theirs. Janet, who was Charcot's most famous pupil, shared his mentor's belief in the hereditary nature of hysteria. But he, far more than Charcot, featured the psychological aspects of hysterical phenomena and felt that his teacher's focus on convulsive symptoms was out of date.[88] Janet focused on how traumatic memories led to the psychological process of dissociation. He posited that some frightening events were so powerful that people could not integrate them into their existing cognitive frameworks. Such frights, or just the ideas of them, led hysterics to split traumatic memories into a separate state of consciousness, one that was outside of their knowledge or control. "The hysterics remembered, but they did not know that they remembered," summarizes historian Michael Roth. Hence, trauma victims had two distinct states of consciousness: one that they knew and another that was hidden from their awareness but persisted in a subconscious, dissociated state. In rare cases, patients developed two or more distinct personalities, none of which was aware of the others.[89]

Janet harshly criticized Freud's focus on the sexual origins of traumatic neuroses.[90] His patients experienced a wide variety of traumas, including accidents, sicknesses, and observing deaths. Unlike the sexually abusive nature of the traumas that Freud would come to emphasize, Janet emphasized how many hysterical symptoms resulted from events such as sleeping beside someone with a gross skin disease, being immersed in freezing water, or unintentionally defecating in front of others. For example, he observed: "One patient has an amaurosis [loss of vision] in her left eye because she has seen a child with scabs on its left eye, and another vomits incessantly because he has nursed a [person with] cancer of the stomach."[91]

Sometimes, even the idea of an event that didn't happen could provoke traumatic symptoms. Janet described a man who was going through one train car to another just as the train was entering a tunnel: "It occurred to him that his left side, which projected, was going to be knocked slantwise and crushed against the arch of the tunnel. This thought caused him to swoon away, but, happily for him, he did not fall on the track, but was taken back inside the carriage, and his left side was not even grazed. In spite of this, he had a left hemiplegy [paralysis of one side of the body]."[92] The intensity of unrecognized memories of these frights produced the personality dissociation that was at the root of traumatic hysteria.

Memories of past traumatic events remained present in a subconscious, disassociated condition but became manifest through hysterical symptoms, including paralysis of limbs, somnambulism, and vomiting. They could have long-term effects on physiological, neurological, and psychic systems, although these impacts were only likely to occur among people with weak central nervous systems.

Like Charcot, Janet often relied on hypnosis to retrieve the hidden memories of his hysterical patients. Uncovering dissociated memories in therapeutic settings could potentially lead patients to assimilate them into consciousness and thereby be cured. Remembering traumas, while a necessary aspect of therapy, was not a sufficient one. Once traumas had been recovered, patients had to be reeducated so that they could deal with their present problems. In contrast to Charcot, however, Janet recognized that the successful recovery of traumatic memories through hypnosis was highly dependent on the degree of patient's vulnerability to therapeutic suggestions. Moreover, far more than Charcot, Janet realized that hysterical symptoms could arise as a result of patients' desires to please their therapists. Because clinicians could exert undue power over their patients, they should take steps, such as increasing the intervals between sessions, to restrict their own influence.[93]

Janet's impact waned after the early years of the twentieth century because his thought (like Charcot's) remained within hereditarian bounds, which emphasized how dissociation was only likely to occur among those who were biologically predisposed to such states. He did not change his views at a time when a new, psychically focused conception of pathology was becoming predominant. In addition, because he did not form a school, he had no intellectual heirs. His thought remained dormant until the 1980s, when feminist therapists rediscovered and used his focus on real, rather than imagined, traumas as a cudgel against Sigmund Freud. The path-breaking models of traumatic hysteria that Freud developed cut the chains of hereditary degeneration that bound both Janet and Charcot and set the stage for a dramatically new view of post-traumatic conditions.

Freud

The work of neurologist and psychoanalyst Sigmund Freud (1856–1939) provided the most significant and lasting historical predecessor of the PTSD diagnosis. His thought regarding trauma is most associated with the conceptions he developed during the 1890s about how repressed sexual disturbances in early childhood led to psychopathology in later life. As a response to the catastrophic events of World War I, Freud also developed another view of trauma (discussed in Chapter 3), which emphasized how the power of contemporaneous, nonsexual, and external shocks produced lasting mental disturbances. Each of these distinct formulations had major consequences for subsequent thinking about PTSD.

Freud's original training in neurology and his brief studies in Paris with Charcot, from October 1885 to February 1886, immersed him in a medical culture that focused on the brain as the seat of mental illness. When he began his initial studies, it was well-recognized that traumatic shocks could produce brain damage and dissociative states. Charcot's and Janet's emphasis on the suppression of memories that followed a trauma had a major impact on Freud. These French predecessors, however, had not shaken the Procrustean bed of heredity that dominated European psychiatry at the time.

Early in his career Freud came to think that brains and minds were much more dynamically interconnected than the prevailing ideas about cerebral localization and heredity would allow. His initial ideas about trauma developed from 1892 to 1896, when he began collaborating with Viennese physician Josef Breuer (1842–1925), who was known for his use of innovative talk therapies for hysterical patients. The hysterics that Breuer treated featured a highly varied array of symptoms—paralysis of limbs, convulsions, tics, vomiting, anorexia, visual and speech disturbances, and hallucinations, among many others.[94] Breuer strove to remove these pathologies by uncovering the buried memories that he believed had produced them. Despite Charcot's recognition that both men and women could develop hysteria, most of Breuer's cases were female. Psychoanalysis was thus born in the study of traumas that befell women. "To a very great extent," observes historian Mark Micale, "the history of hysteria is composed of a body of writing by men about women."[95]

Breuer and Freud viewed hysteria as a post-traumatic neurosis. Although hysterics presented physiological symptoms, Breuer concluded that they were actually symbolic representations of earlier traumas. In their jointly authored *Studies in Hysteria* (1895), they postulated that hysterical symptoms originated in some early, but repressed, trauma. "They are," Breuer and Freud wrote of people with symptoms of hysteria, "valuable theoretically because they have taught us that external events determine the pathology of hysteria to an extent far greater than is known and recognized."[96] Their views about the nature of these events continually changed over the course of the 1890s.

In a marked split with Charcot, Freud and Breuer discarded a hereditarian focus to emphasize how anyone, not just the biologically predisposed, could suffer from the lasting effects of traumas. Childhood traumas caused—not just triggered—neurotic symptoms in later life. Freud and Breuer unambiguously located hysteria in psychological processes. Traumas produced psychic *memories*, which were symbols of those experiences. In contrast to railway accidents, which resulted in symptoms that worked themselves out through conscious reenactments, unconscious memories, ideas, emotions, and desires lay behind the symptoms of hysterical patients.[97] "Hysterics," they memorably wrote, "suffer mainly from reminiscences."[98] Traumatic memories were so intense that patients were unable to consciously assimilate them; they remained repressed within the unconscious so as not to cause mental conflict but later emerged in altered form through the distorted representations of hysterical symptoms. Hysteria, that is, involved physical translations of psychic conflicts that were too painful to remember.[99]

Freud's notion of repression was very similar to Janet's concept of dissociation. In both processes, patients didn't just avoid remembering some trauma; they were *unable* to recollect their traumatic memories. Despite the intense emotions attached to repressed and dissociated memories, both states were unavailable to consciousness. Likewise, neither type displayed the slow fading away that characterized normal processes of memory; instead, memories remained vividly alive in the unconscious. Finally, both repressed and dissociated memories of traumas were not forgotten but endured in the unconscious until they were recovered in therapy. Freud later claimed that "the doctrine of repression is the foundation-stone on which the whole structure of psycho-analysis rests, the most essential part of it."[100]

Freud and Breuer squarely located hysterical symptoms in problems of memory. Normally, memories of past events gradually erode and become less powerful with the passage of time. In hysteria, however, repressed memories of experiences that occurred many years ago remained intense and did not wither away. The resulting symptoms, however, made their demands in the present. And yet, the process that kept memories intense, "unlike other memories of their past lives, are not at the patients' disposal."[101] At the same time as traumatic memories remained in the patient's unconscious, repression led to their conversion into hysterical symptoms. "This can only be explained on the view that these memories constitute an exception in their relation to all the wearing-away processes. . . . *It appears, that is to say, that these memories correspond to traumas that have not been sufficiently abreacted.*"[102] Abreaction—bringing the repressed trauma to consciousness and openly expressing it—deprived the memory of its emotional energy and allowed it to disappear. The powerful, albeit unconscious, impact of past traumas on present symptoms was at the heart of Freud's initial views.

What kinds of trauma produced such powerful, yet repressed, memories? Unlike the variety of traumatic events that Charcot's and Janet's patients displayed, Breuer and Freud traced traumatic events to their origins in sexuality. Breuer emphasized the traumatic impact of sexual events that happened at the time of marriage: "I do not think I am exaggerating when I assert that *the great majority of severe neuroses in women have their origin in the marriage bed.*"[103] Freud, however, rejected Breuer's focus on the traumas that recently married women experienced. He believed that erotically charged events in early childhood or even infancy— for example, sexual abuse, witnessing parental intercourse, or guilt over masturbation—initiated hysterical neurosis.

Freud proposed a radical new thesis: sexual traumas that befell children accounted for every case of hysteria. "The event, the unconscious image of which the patient has retained, is a premature sexual experience with actual stimulation of the genitalia, the result of sexual abuse practiced by another person, and the period of life in which this fateful event occurs is early childhood, up to the age of eight to ten, before the child has attained sexual maturity. *A passive sexual experience before puberty*: this is the specific aetiology of hysteria."[104] Freud insisted that "whatever case and whatever symptom we take as our starting point, *in the end we infallibly come to the realm of sexual experience* as the origin of hysteria."[105] He emphasized that "*these sexual traumas must . . . occur in early childhood (before puberty) and they must consist in actual excitation of the genital organs (coitus-like processes).*"[106] His thesis was so all-encompassing that it could even incorporate railway spine: train crashes led to hysterical symptoms because they recapitulated children's sexual excitement when they engaged in vigorous physical motions.[107] Freud had moved the study of trauma from railway accidents, factory mishaps, or other external hazards to "long forgotten sexual shocks to the nervous system."[108]

Freud's view that actual, but repressed, sexual excitation during childhood caused traumas was short-lived. By 1897 Freud was pursuing a very different line of thought about early traumatic experiences. He was especially interested in the observation that supposedly molested children did not realize that they had undergone traumas when the events occurred. Infants and young children did not know that their sexual excitation was shameful at the time; some of Freud's patients even enjoyed their early sexual stimulation.[109] Only later, usually after entering puberty, did the "traumatic" quality of the event become apparent: "Owing to the changes produced by puberty the memory will exercise a power which was entirely lacking when the experience itself took place: *the memory will produce the same result as if it were an actual event.* We have, so to speak, *the subsequent effect of a sexual trauma.*"[110] While nonsexual early traumas were also repressed, they eventually became inert; the energy released during puberty uniquely impacted early erotic memories.[111]

Freud's intuition that patients in therapy did not recollect the original event, but the memory of the event as they recalled it at a later time, had far-ranging impacts on his conception of trauma: "It is not the experience itself which acts traumatically, but the memory of it when this is re-animated after the subject has entered sexual maturity."[112] Freud had come to believe that when people recall childhood memories they invest them with meanings that stem from their current, as well as their past, states of mind. "Thus," Freud wrote, "what is essentially new about my theory is the thesis that memory is present not once but several times over, that it is laid down in various species of indications."[113]

Freud also thoroughly transformed his early view that adults and older children perpetuated childhood molestations. He admitted that he had misunderstood the nature of patient recollections: "I overestimated the frequency of [infantile seductions by adults] . . . since I was not at this period able to discriminate between the deceptive memories of hysterics concerning their childhood and the memory-traces of actual happenings. I have since learned to unravel many a phantasy of seduction and found it to be an attempt at defence against the memory of sexual activities practiced by the child himself."[114] Freud concluded that memories of sexual abuse stemmed from unconscious fantasies, not from actual sexual assaults. The crucial quality of recollections was not any real sexual stimulation patients had received during early childhood but, instead, how they reacted to their own self-stimulation.

Freud was no longer concerned with reconstructing actual events but instead with exploring wished-for illusions that could not be distinguished from genuine occurrences. In 1899 he coined the term "screen memories," which suggested that memories had components of both fantasy and reality and thus that the memories patients recounted could not be trusted. Their reminiscences were not so much of real sexual experiences as of their unconscious fantasies of sexual desires: "The phantasies possess *psychical* as contrasted to *material* reality, and we gradually learn to understand that *in the world of the neuroses it is psychical reality which is the decisive factor.*"[115]

About a decade later, Freud developed the notion of the Oedipus complex, which referred to the universal sexual longings that very young children have for their opposite sex parents. "Children's sexual wishes," Freud wrote, "awaken very early and . . . a girl's first affection is for her father and a boy's first childish desires are for his mother."[116] The inference was that the later memories of molestations that patients reported did not actually happen but stemmed from their own unconscious desires. From that point until World War I began, Freud became far more interested in patients' subjective longings than in their external experiences. In order to make his initial thesis congruent with his theory of the Oedipus complex, Freud was also forced to alter his contention that strangers, governesses, servants, teachers, older brothers, or other older children perpetuated the sexual traumas that led to the later development of hysterical symptoms.[117] Much later, in 1925, Freud claimed that his early patients had revealed memories of paternal seductions, which actually stemmed from their unconscious erotic attraction to their fathers. Freud had moved the locus of traumas from real events to the unconscious psychic conflicts that influenced patient remembrances.

Treatment

Freud's ideas on how to treat traumas, as well as on their sources, changed considerably over the early phases of his career. At first, he and Breuer located the problems of people who displayed hysteria in their inability to recall the traumatic origins of their symptoms. In their initial writings, they advocated for hypnosis as the treatment of choice for bringing repressed memories to consciousness. On the first page of their 1893 report they stated: "As a rule it is necessary to hypnotize the patient and to arouse his memories under hypnosis of the time at which the symptom made its first appearance."[118]

Breuer's patient, Anna O., provided the model for this work. Like most of Breuer's and Freud's patients, she was a highly educated Jewish woman from a well-off background. While taking care of her dying father, she developed severe symptoms of aphasia, severe headaches, vision disturbances, and paralysis of limbs.[119] She also displayed the amnesia surrounding the trauma behind her symptoms that typified hysterical patients. Although Anna O. presented symptoms that appeared to be physiological, Breuer concluded that they were actually symbolic representations of earlier traumas. Once Breuer had used hypnotism to provoke memories of the forgotten trauma, he claimed that her symptoms disappeared. Breuer concluded his description of this case by noting "the astonishing fact that from beginning to end of the illness all the [symptoms] were permanently removed by being given verbal utterance in hypnosis, and I have only to add an assurance that this was not an invention of mine which I imposed on the patient by suggestion. It took me completely by surprise, and not until symptoms had been got rid of in this way in a whole series of instances did I develop a therapeutic technique out of it."[120]

The implication of Breuer's work was that some active, but unrecognized, part of the mind was implicated in the production of hysterical symptoms. If the failure to remember some trauma led to hysterical symptoms, then getting patients to remember the memory in a hypnotic state should cure the disorder. Once the therapist brought the original experience to consciousness, the unpleasant affect that patients associated with it could be discharged, and the symptoms attached to it would disappear.

Breuer and Freud turned their therapeutic attention toward resurrecting the forgotten past. Therapists must lead their patients to vividly recollect the initial circumstances of the traumatic event and then explicitly discuss their memories with them. Speech allowed the repressed affect to enter normal consciousness, where it lost the emotive force attached to it while memories remained unconscious. Simply talking about repressed symptoms could relieve their debilitating aspects. Once patients had recalled their repressed, early memories, these memories lost their pathological power. "We have seen that hysterical symptoms of the most various kinds which have lasted for many years immediately and permanently disappeared when we had succeeded in bringing clearly to light the memory of the event by which they were provoked and in arousing their accompanying affect, and when the patient had described that event in the greatest possible detail and had put the affect into words."[121] When patients overcame their resistance, clearly recollected both the traumatic event and the accompanying affect, and related it in detail to the therapist, the hysterical symptoms would disappear and never recur.[122] The past must be brought into the present and relived before it could truly remain in the past.

Explorations of repressed memories were long and detailed. This is because patients rarely initially recalled the critical traumatic event, which was actually related to earlier traumatic events that could themselves be traced back to further prior occurrences. "When the scene first revealed does not satisfy our requirements, we say to the patient that this experience does not explain anything, but that there must be hidden behind it an earlier and more significant experience."[123] There was, that is, no simple connection between initial memories of trauma and the bedrock disturbance.

Freud's enthusiasm for hypnosis did not last, and he soon began to emphasize how talk between the patient and the therapist was the central aspect of therapy. He came to believe that the process of transference was the central way to evoke repressed traumatic memories within therapeutic relationships. As a student, Freud had observed the intense erotic desires that Charcot's patients felt toward him. One of Freud's early patients confirmed this experience when she threw her arms around his neck after he had removed her hysterical pains.[124] Freud tried to mobilize the power of such passionate attractions to analysts in the service of therapy. He claimed that patients reexperienced and projected their childhood feelings, especially those toward their parents, onto their therapists in the here and now of the therapy session. The examination of the transference of intense emotions from significant parties in their lives onto their therapists allowed skilled analysts to use what was happening in the present moment as a means of recapturing, however imperfectly, the past traumatic memories that were at the root of the patient's current problems. Freud believed that transference was a more powerful technique than hypnosis; in contrast to the minority of patients who are hypnotizable, virtually all patients want to please their therapists.

Both hypnosis and talk therapies centering on transference raise questions about the role of therapists in not just uncovering traumatic memories but of actually creating these memories. Many critics now believe that Freud *implanted* rather than simply described the memories he sought to disarm.[125] Most notoriously, Freud essentially bullied one of his most famous patients, Dora, to admit that her denials that she was in love with one of her father's friends actually indicated that she did love him: "If this 'No,' instead of being regarded as the expression of an impartial judgement . . . is ignored, and if work is continued, the first evidence soon begins to appear that in such a case 'No' signifies the desired 'Yes.' "[126] Another of Freud's patients, Elisabeth von R., recollected that he tried "to persuade me that I was in love with my brother-in-law, but that wasn't really so."[127] Freud was particularly unshakeable in his belief about the importance of the Oedipus complex as underlying traumatic memories. Patients' desires to please their clinicians can lead them to produce the same dynamics that they think their therapists expect them to have.

As early as 1896, the prominent psychiatrist Richard von Krafft-Ebing accused Freud of using suggestion to elicit traumatic memories.[128] Freud's friend, Wilhelm Fliess, also observed that Freud attributed his own theories about the traumatic origins of hysteria to the minds of his patients.[129] Especially after Freud had come to regard memory as a subjective process that did not mirror actual events, therapeutic suggestion became an outsized source of what patients recollected. Just as Charcot's hysterical patients produced the symptoms they thought he wanted to see, Freud's patients could easily construct whatever narrative seemed most appealing to him.

Freud himself always denied any role of suggestion in his treatments: "I do not believe even now that I forced the seduction-fantasies on my patients, that I 'suggested' them," he stated in 1925.[130] Yet, his own reports about his technique lend credence to the view that he induced rather than discovered the unconscious memories he uncovered: "But the fact is that patients never relate these histories spontaneously, and never suddenly offer, in the course of the treatment, the complete recollection of such a scene to the physician. The mental image of the premature sexual experience is recalled only when most energetic pressure is exerted by the analytic procedure, against strong resistance; so that the recollection has to be extracted bit by bit from the patients."[131] Indeed, Freud noted: "Before they come for analysis the patients know nothing about these scenes [of early childhood abuse]." He went on to say that "only the strongest compulsion of the treatment can induce them to embark on a reproduction of them."[132]

The role of clinical suggestion became especially important once Freud had come to see traumas as products of psychic forces that are unamenable to direct observation rather than actual events that might have some external source of validation. In contrast to much medical thought at the time, however, Freud did not think patients were malingerers, who consciously profited from their symptoms; instead, repression brought about purely psychic benefits that exceeded the costs of revealing their traumatic origins.

After the turn of the nineteenth century, Freud's attention moved from his early focus on the traumas leading to hysterical symptoms to how unconscious processes manifested themselves in dreams, jokes, slips of the tongue, sexuality, and various psychic defenses. Between 1900 and 1914 psychoanalytic theory and practice revolved around the conflicts between the conscious and the unconscious and between the libido and the ego. On the eve of World War I, traumas no longer held center stage in Freud's theories or therapeutic encounters. The bloodbath of this war led Freud to develop a conception of trauma that thoroughly diverged from his earlier views.

CONCLUSION

Three different pathways created the recognition of traumatic events as sources of mental disorders in the last half of the nineteenth century. The terrors of combat during the American Civil War led many soldiers to develop and record lasting psychic disturbances. Because traumatic psychic symptoms rarely led to compensation at the time and because clinicians had no conceptions of these conditions, their emergence during and after the war likely indicated genuine disturbances. However, extant medical and cultural interpretations did not provide a disease framework for these mental impairments.

The explicit notion that external events could produce lasting psychic memories of trauma emerged in the context of widespread mechanized accidents. These traumatic symptoms often emerged immediately after intense stressors, although some seemed to become more intense with the passage of time. Unlike the uncompensated lingering conditions of soldiers at the time, victims of train crashes and other accidents could bring lawsuits against corporations. The recognition of traumatic disorders thus emerged as controversial products of litigation and alleged secondary gains.

Psychiatry provided the third conduit for the emergence of traumatic mental disorders. While Charcot and Janet emphasized the lasting impacts of traumas, their thought remained embedded within hereditarian thinking, which viewed external shocks more as triggers than as causes of psychic symptoms. Freud then directed the focus of traumatic attention toward the unconscious psychic underpinnings of childhood sexual abuse and desires. His thinking turned psychiatry away from its focus on biologically grounded hereditarian theories to, first, actual and, then, to imagined psychic shocks. However, Freud was never able to show that the conditions he treated were grounded in either patients' actual problems or their fantasies as opposed to his own suggestions.

The late nineteenth-century's emphasis on the lasting impact of traumatic experiences during early life, especially those befalling girls and women, was inapplicable to the catastrophic destruction and psychic trauma that accompanied the wars of the twentieth century. The horrors of World War I turned public and professional attention to men who faced in real time the devastating psychic consequences of combat and its aftermath.

CHAPTER THREE

The Psychic Wounds of Combat

> I was still mentally and nervously organized for war; shells used to come bursting on my bed at mid-night even when Nancy was sharing it with me; strangers in day-time would assume the faces of friends who had been killed.
>
> Robert Graves, *Goodbye to All That*

> The past is gone, Tom thought, and I will not brood about it. I've got to be tough. I am not the type to have a nervous breakdown. I can't afford it. I have too many responsibilities. This is a time of peace, and I will forget about the war.
>
> Sloan Wilson, *The Man in the Gray Flannel Suit*

The issue of post-traumatic stress posed an immediate, and enormous, problem for the various militaries involved in World War I. When the war began in 1914, traumas were already well established, if highly contentious, causes of psychological damage. Yet, the dominant existing frameworks for understanding traumas were not well-suited for dealing with the massive numbers of psychic casualties the war had produced.

Psychiatrists at the time focused on the unconscious impacts of childhood traumas among its mostly female clientele. Some, such as Charcot and Janet, emphasized the role of preexisting biological vulnerabilities. Others, including Freud, stressed how repressed memories of early sexual fantasies led to later hysterical symptoms. The emphasis on the lasting psychic impacts of traumas from the distant past and on unconscious processes were not promising ways of explaining the huge number of men who suffered from the real, contemporaneous shocks of war.

Moreover, the extant psychiatric views could not account for the confrontation between the power of extreme circumstances to produce psychic breakdowns and the influence of social norms that regarded psychic casualties as unmanly. Medical conceptions of war-related traumas struggled to emerge from the tight grip that cultural standards of appropriate male behavior held over responses to the terrors of combat. Beliefs that expressions of distress associated with trauma represented weakness or cowardice persisted throughout this period.

The concern with the psychic impact of railway and industrial accidents provided a more relevant framework for understanding how external shocks could produce brain changes and resulting psychic symptoms. It raised the possibility that traumas led to psychological disturbances among previously normal victims. Nevertheless, many physicians, who claimed that such shocks only triggered symptoms in already predisposed individuals, vigorously opposed this idea. In addition, the disputes over railway spine embedded traumas within a legal framework in which the interests of plaintiffs and defendants sharply conflicted. This led many observers to doubt the motives of traumatized victims, who they felt simulated their symptoms in order to obtain compensation. Questions about malingering were of particular concern to the military, which regarded malingerers as a serious challenge to morale and the need to maintain ample manpower.

From 1914 through 1945 and beyond, issues surrounding the psychic devastation of the wars and their aftermath became a prominent theme in medicine and the general culture. During this era clinicians attended to the immediate and lasting impacts of combat on psychic disturbances. This emphasis turned psychiatry away from the inner dynamics related to early childhood traumas and toward the role of extreme, contemporaneous, and external stressors as causes of mental disorders. It also moved the clinical focus from the problems of traumatized females to the wartime and postwar experiences of male combatants. Because governments, not private insurers or individuals and their families, were responsible for the welfare of damaged combatants, they became central players in definitions of and responses to traumatic events.

WORLD WAR I

As in the Civil War, the vast majority of combatants in the First World War were conscripts, not professionals. They faced new forms of conflict, which involved a combination of the massive use of high explosives with long periods of trench warfare. Battles often involved periods of passive waiting for artillery shells to explode when men could neither fight nor flee. The introduction of poison gas also provided a new, highly lethal form of battlefield terror. Unsurprisingly, the result was a huge and unprecedented number of psychiatric casualties.

Shell Shock

When World War I began, military physicians and psychiatrists were thoroughly unprepared to deal with the unprecedented quantity of psychic casualties that arose among combatants. Seemingly out of the blue, the initial artillery bombardments in 1914 resulted in an unexpected epidemic of men who developed hysterical deafness, muteness, blindness, paralysis of limbs, and violent tremors. By the end of the war the British, French, and American forces had suffered about 800,000, 800,000, and 100,000 traumatic neuroses, respectively.[1]

At first, medical professionals reworked theories associated with railway spine to explain symptoms as products of the relationship between exploding artillery shells and resulting physical brain lesions.[2] In 1915 Charles Myers (1873–1946), an English military doctor, coined the term "shell-shock" to characterize this condition.[3] Although Myers later admitted that the term was unsuitable for traumatic symptoms, he initially believed that the physical force of exploding shells led to hysterical symptoms—to uncontrollable tremors and twitches, nightmares, serious confusion, delirium, and amnesia: "There were descriptions of cases with starting eyes, violent tremors, a look of terror, and blue, cold extremities. Some were deaf and some were dumb; others were blind or paralyzed."[4] Such symptoms were more common among ordinary soldiers than among officers, who were more likely to show neurasthenic-like symptoms, including depression, anxiety, and insomnia.[5]

It soon became apparent, however, that shell shock almost never occurred among soldiers who were actually wounded by shells.[6] Instead, almost all "shell-shocked" soldiers had no physical wounds but suffered from fear-related psychological conditions.[7] "Shell-shock" was an inappropriate label for the vast majority of sufferers who were mentally, but not physically, disabled. As Myers explained twenty years after the war had ended, shell shock does "not depend for [its] causation on the physical force (or the chemical effects) of the bursting shell. [It] may also occur when the soldier is remote from the exploding missile, provided that he be subject to an emotional disturbance or mental strain sufficiently severe."[8]

The resemblance of many symptoms of shell shock to hysteria was embarrassing. Despite Charcot's appreciation that men as well as women could develop hysteria, "Hysteria was something that happened to women. Doctors tried to find another name for it so as to spare their patients the shame of being called hysterics."[9] Myers recognized the similarities of soldiers' presentations to hysteria, but he didn't want to associate them with a female-related disorder, so he called it "shell-shock." This label provided soldiers with an honorable, organically based injury that was tied to the conditions of combat rather than to psychic weakness or cowardice. Conceptions of shell shock not only dominated military psychiatry for the duration of the war but also became a major theme about combat experiences in popular culture.[10]

As psychic casualties mounted, military physicians had no choice but to recognize the similarities of the symptoms they treated with the hysterical displays that Charcot, Freud, and others had observed. They faced the difficult task of explaining how combat or the fears associated with the possibility of entering combat could so closely resemble the conditions of women who presumably suffered from traumas they had experienced as children.[11]

Shell shock fundamentally challenged the gender norms that dominated the military. Conceptions of masculinity and warfare had been inseparable for thousands of years. Service in World War I was viewed as essential for establishing manhood. Historian John Kinder observes how "US military recruiters made warrior masculinity a central part of their enlistment campaigns." Harold Peat, who became the most famous spokesman for disabled soldiers, proclaimed that his pain and suffering had made him "more of a man."[12] Most officers and politicians, as well as the general public, felt that men afflicted with shell shock had lost control of their emotions and succumbed to their fears; they were unmanly, effeminate, weak, and cowardly. Shell-shocked soldiers had not just failed the test that war presented to manliness but had also assumed passive patient roles, which were more suitable for women than for men. In this view, such cowardly reactions must be met with harsh discipline, both to prevent secondary gains from the sick role and to set an example that other soldiers would not want to follow.

Explaining Shell Shock

Medical professionals could not reach a consensus regarding the causes of war-related psychic traumas. A sharp debate arose that reproduced the dispute among neurologists and physicians about railway spine. One group of military psychiatrists focused on hereditary factors, as well as the possibility of malingering, to explain the conditions of shell-shocked soldiers. They continued to view psychic casualties as products of degeneration and constitutional weakness.[13] Most traumatized soldiers, they emphasized, had preexisting conditions of neurosis, psychosis, alcoholism, or neurasthenia, so the war was at best a precipitating, but not a causal, factor for their symptoms.

Many military doctors and psychiatrists focused on these personal vulnerabilities and downplayed the role of external conditions connected to the war. They felt that any condition caused by war trauma itself should be easily and quickly curable and would not have lasting effects. In contrast, chronic conditions likely stemmed from predisposing factors that were unrelated to war experiences or from malingering to avoid the dangers of the battlefield or to obtain a pension after the war had ended. These physicians noted that physically wounded soldiers, who did not need an excuse to avoid further combat, did not develop psychic impairments, which indicated to them that psychic symptoms represented attempts to evade combat.[14] "The psychogenic theory of war neurosis became dominant to a large extent because it allowed the army neither to release war hysterics from duty, nor to pay them compensation," historian Esther Fischer-Homberger concludes.[15]

A contrasting view focused on how the nature of battle itself caused shell shock. One version of this explanation, exemplified by Myers's initial portrayal, stressed how the loud sounds of exploding shells led to changes in the brain. The most influential proponent of this focus was German neurologist Hermann Oppenheim.[16] Oppenheim noted the similarity of war traumas to industrial accidents because both were caused by minute changes of brain molecules that were unrelated to psychic causes. A second type of environmental causation discarded this organic perspective and emphasized how an accumulation of stress could lead any soldier, whether predisposed or not, to break down. British anatomist Grafton Elliot Smith and psychologist Tom Pear contended that World War I "has shown us one indisputable fact, that a psychoneurosis may be produced in almost anyone if only his environment be made 'difficult' enough for him. It has warned us that the pessimistic, helpless appeal to heredity, so common in the case of insanity must [be abandoned]. . . . In the causation of the psychoneuroses, heredity undoubtedly counts, but social and material environment count infinitely more."[17]

Similar debates took place among psychoanalysts. This group had a difficult time reconciling their focus on unconscious internal mental processes with the role of external environmental traumas. Some analysts, most prominently Karl Abraham and Sándor Ferenczi, posited that most psychic casualties of the war had already been prone to neuroses before the war. They emphasized how soldiers who were neurotic when they entered military service responded differently to the terrors of combat from those who had not previously been psychically disturbed.[18] Many American observers also faulted "hasty medical examiners [who] had passed for induction men whose mental stability was questionable."[19] In this view, predisposed soldiers accounted for the bulk of subsequent combat and postwar neuropsychiatric cases.

Other dynamically oriented practitioners, most notably British psychiatrist W. H. R. Rivers (1864–1922), focused on the conflict between the instinct to survive and the duty to one's group.[20] Rivers associated hysterical symptoms with the passive, immobile, and helpless situations of soldiers in trenches. Such symptoms arose because men were intensely fearful and yet were unable to flee combat because they also felt that they must uphold ideals of honor, duty, and patriotism. This unresolvable situation led soldiers to unconsciously displace their fears onto hysterical symptoms and thus escape from an intolerable conflict. Because sufferers were not aware of these processes, Rivers and other advocates of the importance of psychodynamic processes did not believe that traumatized soldiers should be held accountable for their symptoms. Moreover, when put under enough stress, all men could develop combat-related neuroses.

Freud himself fundamentally revised his theory in response to the massive psychic traumas of World War I. The war posed a basic challenge to his conception of traumatic neuroses: childhood sexual traumas, whether real or imagined, seemingly had no power to account for why so many soldiers succumbed to the terrors of the battlefield. Combatants clearly had to worry about real, present dangers, not repressed memories of early sexual desires. Yet, many soldiers developed the same sorts of paralysis of limbs, muteness, deafness, and blindness that characterized some hysterical female patients. The war forced Freud to turn his attention from the psychoneuroses that were products of early experiences to the actual neuroses that resulted from contemporaneous shocks.[21]

Freud thoroughly revised his view of traumatic neuroses.[22] In *Beyond the Pleasure Principle* (1920), he elaborated on the distinction between war neuroses, which stemmed from external dangers, and neuroses of peace, in which people defended themselves from internal threats. Anticipating the stressor-oriented post-traumatic stress disorder diagnosis in the *DSM-III*, he developed the idea that traumas were marked by powerful, unexpected mental excitation that broke through the protective shields that individuals used to maintain their psychic equilibrium.[23] People who anticipated a traumatic experience were unlikely to develop neuroses. Those who were unprepared for the violent event and so were surprised by it, however, were flooded with more frightening stimuli than they were able to master and accommodate. Traumatic neuroses thus resulted from external, unanticipated, unpleasant, and overwhelming experiences in the present, not in the past. Crucially, Freud's later view focused on the overwhelming impact of the traumatic shock itself, not on any predisposing personality factor.

Freud's revised conception of trauma also foreshadowed the focus on reexperiencing the traumatic situation that emerged many years later in the *DSM-III* PTSD diagnosis.[24] Freud wrote: "The traumatic neuroses give a clear indication that a fixation to the traumatic accident lives at their root. These patients regularly repeat the traumatic situation in their dreams; where hysteriform attacks occur that admit of an analysis, we find that the attack corresponds to a complete transplanting of the patient into the traumatic situation. It is as though these patients had not yet finished with the traumatic situation, as though they were still faced by it as an immediate task which has not been dealt with; and we take this view quite seriously."[25] This passage antedates the

DSM-III's criteria, which require at least one of "recurrent and intrusive recollections of the event; recurrent dreams of the event; and sudden acting or feeling as if the traumatic event were reoccurring."[26] Conversely, it turns away from Freud's earlier views, which featured the importance of repression as a defense against recalling traumatic memories.

Freud's observation of wartime traumas also led him to thoroughly revise his theory of dreams and the unconscious. He observed that, in contrast to their waking lives, in which people tried to avoid thinking about traumas, in dreams traumatized soldiers were repeatedly taken back to the traumatic situation.[27] His prior theory that dreams were forms of wish fulfillment could not explain this phenomenon: "Now dreams occurring in traumatic neuroses have the characteristic of repeatedly bringing the patient back into the situation of his accident, a situation from which he wakes up in another fright. This astonishes people far too little."[28] He concluded that soldiers continued to experience traumas such as exploding shells in their dreams as attempts to retrospectively master and stabilize their inner lives, not as ways to obtain pleasure.[29] Psychic repetitions of the event represented attempts to anticipate, react to, and assimilate the trauma so that healing could occur. "It is as though these patients had not yet finished with the traumatic situation, as though they were still faced by it as an immediate task which has not been dealt with," Freud summarized.[30]

Although Freud struggled to integrate his insights about traumatic neuroses into his broader theory, the origins of current conceptions of PTSD are found in his response to World War I. His focus on powerful external shocks in turn had a major impact on Abram Kardiner, the most prominent theorist of war trauma during World War II and, through Kardiner and his heirs, on the PTSD diagnosis in *DSM-III*.

Responses to Shell Shock

The treatment of shell-shocked soldiers elicited considerable controversy. At the beginning of the war, doctors tried many therapies—hypnosis, drugs, psychotherapy, electroshock, and discipline—but none was successful. Following the view of most military physicians and psychiatrists, the army typically treated shell-shocked soldiers as cowardly malingerers. Officers initially reacted very harshly to shell-shocked soldiers, including the use of firing squads. At the extreme, British neurologist H. W. Hills observed that some of his colleagues felt that "if a man lets his comrades down he ought to be shot. If he's a loony, so much the better."[31] As casualties mounted over the course of the war, the need to keep soldiers in combat became more pressing. Perceived malingering threatened both manpower and morale. British psychiatrist Lewis Yealland became the representative of electroshock and disciplinary therapies that emphasized fast, brutal, and shaming techniques. In Germany, too, a number of neurologists applied strong electrical shocks to overcome patient resistance to reentering combat.[32]

Over the course of the war, many psychiatrists came to adopt attitudes of sympathetic understanding for victims of shell shock.[33] A number of this group used psychotherapeutic methods to disarm memories of combat-related traumas. Most notably, the psychodynamically oriented Rivers found that some aspects of Freud's early theories explained how suppressed terror came to be converted into physical symptoms. Rivers emphasized the importance of recovering suppressed memories of the combat trauma through techniques that brought to the surface the unconscious conflicts that he believed underlay symptoms. Rivers and like-minded psychiatrists used hypnosis, dream interpretation, and transference to treat shell-shocked patients.[34] Charles Myers, too, used hypnosis to recover lost memories of the trauma, restore them to consciousness, and, presumably, lead them to disappear.[35] But, even these more compassionate physicians and psychiatrists confronted a quandary: if their patients recovered they would reenter combat and face retraumatization or death.

A third, and ultimately the most influential, group promoted the idea that the treatment of shell-shocked soldiers should be prompt, simple, and occur near the front lines.[36] What came to be called "PIE" treatment—proximity to the battlefield, immediate response, and expectation of quick recovery—became a standard intervention among the French, British, and American forces.[37] Physicians tried not to remove psychic casualties to distant hospitals, where they feared symptoms would stabilize. Instead, they set up field hospitals near battlefields where combatants could receive rest and reassurance.[38] American psychiatrists, led by Thomas Salmon, also used basic responses toward afflicted soldiers that involved healthy food, enough sleep and exercise, and encouragement of positive attitudes toward resuming normal roles.[39]

The variety of therapeutic positions meant that luck often determined the actual response a shell-shocked soldier received: "Depending on the circumstances, a shell-shocked soldier might earn a wound stripe and a pension . . . be shot for cowardice, or simply be told to pull himself together by his medical office and sent back to duty," historian Ben Shephard concludes.[40] Clinicians never resolved the intermingling of psychiatric theories, military discipline, and traditional codes of masculinity in responses to shell-shocked combatants.

The First World War resulted in a much greater awareness of the importance of external causes of psychic traumas. Despite its numerous interpretations, shell shock provided a new framework for understanding the psychological casualties of combat for the military, the state, physicians, society, and soldiers themselves. It also led to the widespread use of short-term treatments for traumatic symptoms. Perhaps most importantly, it led the notion of trauma to enter the collective consciousness of Western cultures.

Postwar Problems

The end of the war did not resolve the problem of how to deal with shell-shocked soldiers; indeed, it worsened it. By 1920 almost all European countries faced widespread unemployment, poverty, housing shortages, and falling living standards. Psychically impaired ex-servicemen became a widespread and familiar phenomenon. More than 300,000 German and more than 400,000 British veterans were estimated to have persistent psychological wounds from the war.[41] Their high visibility led shell shock to enter post-war culture as well as medicine and psychiatry.

Shell shock was especially noticeable in English culture, where it became a dominant theme in poetry, novels, plays, and films.[42] A prominent example was Siegfried Sassoon's memoir, *Sherston's Progress*, which emphasized how shell shock might only take effect long after the initial combat experience: "Shell-shock. How many a brief bombardment had its long-delayed after-effect in the minds of these survivors, many of whom had looked at their companions and laughed while inferno did its best to destroy them. Not then was their evil hour, but now; now in the sweating suffocation of nightmare, in paralysis of limbs, in the stammering of dislocated speech."[43] A major English postwar literary figure, Robert Graves, noted his PTSD-like condition (which, like those of many officers, was officially labeled "neurasthenia"): "I was still mentally and nervously organized for War. Shells used to come bursting on my bed at midnight, even though Nancy [his wife] shared it with me; strangers in daytime would assume the faces of friends who had been killed. . . . My family . . . did not know quite how to treat me."[44] Virginia Wolff's *Mrs. Dalloway* depicted a war veteran, Septimus Smith, who displays characteristic PTSD symptoms of numbness, intrusive memories of traumatic combat experiences, and hallucinations of the death of a comrade: "The dead were with him. 'Evans, Evans!' [a dead comrade killed in the war] he cried."[45]

American sociologist Willard Waller recognized that almost all veterans carried memories of jumbled emotions of "fear, horror, guilt and anger."[46] They were subject to queer moods and tempers, loss of control, and bitterness. During the day they experienced pronounced startle reactions, especially after noises that sounded like shells, while evil dreams haunted them at night. One war correspondent noted: "Something was wrong. They put on civilian clothes again and looked to their mothers and wives very much like the young men who had gone to business in the peaceful days before August 1914. But they had not come back the same men. Something had altered in them. They were subject to sudden moods and queer tempers, fits of profound depression alternating with a restless drive for pleasure."[47] Although the term "shell-shock" had been discredited, no alternative psychiatric label replaced it. Veterans who entered treatment systems tended to be grouped into existing psychoneurotic conditions, namely, neurasthenia, hysteria, or psychasthenia.[48]

American psychiatrist Abram Kardiner (1891–1981) wrote the most important postwar book about the psychological damage of World War I veterans, although it wasn't published until 1941, when the Second World War was already under way. Kardiner was psychodynamically oriented, pursuing Freud's later insights about the relationship between external events and traumatic neuroses.[49] He generally adopted Freud's position that combat neuroses were the result of abrupt changes in the external environment leading to extreme degrees of physiological arousal that individuals had insufficient resources to master. Kardiner coined the term "physioneurosis" to emphasize the joint biological and psychological components of combat-related conditions. Victims tried to gain emotional distance from their trauma at the same time as their bodies reacted to external reminders of their trauma with involuntary, often extreme, states of physical arousal.

Physioneuroses could involve a great variety of symptoms: repetitive tics, feelings of reliving the traumatic situation, tremors, paralysis of limbs, irritability, tendencies to aggression and violence, sexual impotence, anxiety, phobias, fatigue, and sleep difficulties.[50] Hysterical disturbances of gait and speech disorders, such as stammering, aphonias, and mutism, were especially common.[51] In addition, Kardiner's patients often had no recollection or incomplete memories of the trauma itself. Although many of them actively strove to avoid remembering traumatic events during their waking lives, as Freud had observed, they typically relived them in their dreams.[52]

Kardiner emphasized how immediate treatment was necessary so that symptoms wouldn't become chronic and exploited by individuals for secondary gains, noting that "the traumatic neuroses fared badly in psychoanalysis."[53] He also rarely used hypnosis because he felt it prevented the recognition of the connection between the trauma and resulting symptoms. While Kardiner occasionally employed sedatives, he downplayed the importance of drugs and regarded them as not "even an important accessory" to therapy.[54] Instead, following the basic principles of PIE treatments, he claimed that "an atmosphere of rest and assurance are of the greatest importance."[55]

In contrast to other dynamically oriented therapists, Kardiner did not think it was wise to allow patients to recall images connected with the original trauma.[56] Instead, clinicians should encourage them to adjust to their current reality. Recovery depended on a combination of internal resources, relationships with primary groups, and the presence of strong sources of social support. Kardiner claimed that between half and 90 percent of traumatic neuroses could be prevented through such simple means.[57] "By far the most important forensic aspect of the traumatic neurosis is that it should not be allowed to become stabilized," he concluded.[58] Pensions would become the most important factor leading psychic traumas to persist.

Pensions

A major postwar concern, echoing the aftermath of the Civil War, was the impact of shell shock on government finances. Compensation was a particularly problematic response to combat trauma because, in contrast to the neuroses of peacetime, when insurance companies were liable for damages, governments were responsible for reimbursing sufferers of war neuroses. While insurers had an inherent interest in denying or minimizing compensation, states faced special pressures to reward damaged veterans. As Waller observed: "The veteran is always a powerful political force, for good or evil, because . . . [h]e has fought for the flag and absorbed some of the *mana*. He is sacred. He is covered with pathos and immune from criticism."[59] Overgenerous compensatory policies could, however, ruin government finances as well as stabilize symptoms.

Widespread apprehension developed after World War I that

the lingering psychological effects of traumas would produce unsustainable numbers of claims for disability pensions. General suspicion of chronic psychological casualties prevailed. The question of who was a "deserving" beneficiary of financial compensation came to the fore: How could ex-soldiers who had suffered genuine psychic traumas in combat and therefore truly merited compensation be distinguished from those who simulated psychic wounds to escape the battlefield or to seek unmerited rewards?

Increasing pension costs for treating war neurotics created deep alarm in many nations. In the decade following the war, more than 100,000 British ex-servicemen applied for pensions due to shell shock.[60] By 1918 about 6 percent of British pensions had been awarded for this condition (an additional 11 percent were awarded for heart problems, many of which were psychosomatic in nature).[61] The problem of secondary gain from chronic shell shock was paramount. A British commission that investigated the implications of shell shock for postwar society concluded "that this class of case excited more general interest, attention, and sympathy than any other, so much so that it became a most desirable complaint from which to suffer."[62] A committee formed in 1939 to investigate the problem of pensions for shell-shocked veterans concluded: "There can be no doubt that in the overwhelming proportion of cases, these patients succumb to 'shock' because they get something out of it."[63]

German psychiatrists expected that traumatic neuroses among people who were not otherwise predisposed to become neurotic would rapidly clear.[64] Therefore, soldiers with chronic conditions must have some preexisting infirmity that made them already prone to become neurotic. One psychiatric advisor to the War Ministry claimed that his review of 463 neurasthenic pensioners showed that: "57% had served at home only and . . . 59% had a pre-war history of neurotic illness or tendency."[65] Other German psychiatrists thought that shell shock victims were cowards and malingerers.[66]

In the United States, after the initial victory parades, veterans returned to a "hostile social climate marked by widespread unemployment, political intolerance, and growing ambivalence about the costs of American victory."[67] At the end of 1919, psychological cases constituted about 40 percent of all hospitalized veterans.[68] As in Europe, concern grew over the pension costs and widespread fraud that claims of war-related psychic damage might involve.

Two veterans' organizations, the American Legion and the Disabled American Veterans of the World War, were major advocacy groups. Their goal was to change perceptions of war neurosis and to make the federal government responsible for mental health care. These groups took special interest in shell-shocked veterans, portraying mentally disturbed soldiers as "honorable men overwhelmed by the horrors of war."[69] They directed their lobbying efforts for veterans toward obtaining better pensions, generous civil service preferences, and expanded eligibility for federal programs. They were often successful: "Legionnaires and comrades carved out a privileged legal status for war-disabled vets, one that accorded them monetary and institutional benefits superseding those of all other US citizens."[70]

The lobbying efforts of these groups led the federal government to recognize the need to deal with disabled vets on an ongoing and permanent basis. Rehabilitation programs that strove to make incapacitated veterans useful citizens who could work and thus be saved from unmanly forms of dependency became firmly embedded in US policy: "The rehabilitation movement of World War I marked a major turning point in the development of the veterans' welfare state. It institutionalized the federal government's obligation to restore disabled veterans to a state of masculine productivity."[71] By 1923 close to 1 million soldiers had applied for disability benefits.[72] The expansion of eligibility criteria led the number of pensioners to soar by 866 percent between 1919 and 1929.[73] By 1932 expenditures on World War I veterans' benefits—$581 million in that year—was the single largest cost to the federal government.[74] Between the two world wars, the United States spent nearly a billion dollars on veterans' psychiatric illnesses.[75]

Some backlash developed as neuropsychiatric casualties threatened to swamp government resources. Waller stated a common view that pensions could make recovery impossible: "Pensions may thus do positive harm to the psychoneurotic." Indeed, he noted, "It may come about that a man makes his living by having a war neurosis," and he said that "the fakes, the chisellers, the fraudulent wounded who flourish after every war will never hesitate to press their claims."[76] Social historian Dixon Wecter likewise warned that "being a veteran, among certain groups, was in danger of degenerating into just another racket."[77] Tensions also remained between efforts to broaden pensions and traditional codes of masculinity, which connected dependency with weakness and feminization. " 'Real men' did not complain when things turned bad, and they certainly did not badger the government for handouts"; they were expected "to keep quiet, forget the past, and move forward with their lives," historian John Kinder observes.[78]

By the 1930s economic decline, mass unemployment, and decreasing tax revenues made the support of disabled veterans difficult. For example, in Great Britain, 40,000 World War I soldiers, many of whom had never seen combat, were still receiving pensions in 1939.[79] Because the continued reception of a pension depended on maintaining symptoms, many observers feared that pensions did not promote recovery but turned men into chronic neurotics. A more moralistic, judgmental climate emerged as the psychically disabled were associated with pathological dependency and compromised masculinity.[80] The dilemma of how the state could compensate worthy soldiers without creating chronic conditions endured throughout the twentieth century and beyond.

WORLD WAR II

Despite the widespread attention that shell shock received during and after the First World War, the various militaries involved in World War II were not ready for the enormous numbers of psychic casualties that emerged almost immediately after the war began. For example, the British had not anticipated the huge number of shell-shocked troops among the evacuees from Dunkirk in 1940 that had to be hospitalized.[81] The American military, as well, was unprepared for the psychiatric casualties that the entry into World War II created. In 1941 the entire psychiatric staff of the armed services comprised only 25 members. Over the course of the war, a wholesale transformation occurred as psychiatric casualties and their treatment became a major focus of the war effort. By the war's end, some 2,400 physicians were engaged in psychiatric activities.[82]

The American Experience of Screening

The American military's initial attempt to deal with the threat of mental disturbance involved implementing a widespread program to identify and prevent the mentally ill from entering the armed services. This screening was based on the assumption that, first, only biologically or psychologically predisposed individuals would break down in combat, and, second, that it was possible to recognize these persons before they entered military service.

At first, the armed services had great faith that psychically vulnerable soldiers could be detected and kept out of service. Noted psychiatrist Harry Stack Sullivan (1892–1949), who believed that a fifteen-minute interview could distinguish which recruits would be susceptible to breakdowns, developed the early screening protocols.[83] These instruments used very broad criteria, including such traits as shyness, discontent, irritability, alcohol and tobacco use, and homosexual tendencies.[84] Overall, their use resulted in the rejection as psychologically unfit for military service of nearly two million potential soldiers, about 12 percent of all recruits. An additional three-quarters of a million draftees were separated from the military for mental defects after they had entered service but before they entered combat.[85]

Screening programs quickly broke down under the weight of the massive numbers of men excluded from entering the military, the wide divergences in results across different sites and examiners, and the inability to develop an effective screening tool. Most importantly, screening instruments could not predict who would become a psychiatric casualty of combat. Postwar studies that compared rates of impairment before and after screening had been discontinued showed that this technique did not accurately identify which soldiers would break down in combat.[86]

During the war, more than a million American servicemen entered psychiatric facilities, most for combat-related psychoneuroses. It soon became apparent that the actual reasons for their psychiatric breakdowns had little to do with the sorts of predispositions that screening instruments had been designed to identify. In addition, the enormous number of men who were rejected from duty because of their supposed mental problems threatened the military's increasing need for manpower. By 1943, the military had come to place a very low priority on screening recruits for psychiatric problems.[87]

Psychic Casualties

More than a million psychiatric admissions to British hospitals occurred during the war years, with rates as high as 25 percent in combat units.[88] The American military suffered equally high numbers of psychiatric casualties. By the end of 1942, mental disorders accounted for more than a quarter of all hospital admissions among US soldiers. In the most intense fighting, such as the bloody battle for Guadalcanal in 1942, some 40 percent of the wounded were deemed casualties for psychiatric reasons. The 112,000 psychic breakdowns among American soldiers in 1943 almost equaled the number of men who were drafted in that year.[89] During the most intense battles in Europe during 1944, up to three-quarters of soldiers suffered psychic breakdowns.[90] Over the course of the war, more than a million American military personnel were admitted to psychiatric facilities.[91] This rate was between two and three times greater than in World War I.[92] Overall, psychiatric reasons accounted for about half of all medical discharges from the American armed forces.[93]

A notable aspect of World War II psychic casualties was the almost complete absence of the hysterical symptoms that had marked so many soldiers during the previous world war.[94] Instead, combatants typically displayed the anxious and depressive symptoms that were comparable to the conditions that outpatient psychiatrists and physicians were seeing in the general culture.[95] Military psychiatrist Roy Grinker found that the five most common psychic symptoms were restlessness, irritability or aggression, fatigue on arising, sleep difficulties, and anxiety.[96] None of the nineteen most prevalent symptoms he listed had any resemblance to the hysterical symptoms that characterized breakdowns during World War I. This curious phenomenon might indicate that soldiers, like psychiatric patients in general, produce the symptoms that medical personnel and their culture expect them to display.[97]

The absence of cases resembling shell shock led to a thoroughgoing change in terminology. Very general terms such as "combat neurosis," "combat exhaustion," or "war neurosis" replaced what had previously been called "shell-shock." Just as the label "PTSD" would later do, each of these terms made an intrinsic connection between an external stressor and a resultant psychic disturbance. "Out of these [combat] experiences came an awareness that social and situational determinants of behavior were more important than the assets and liabilities of individuals involved in coping with wartime stress and strain," one government report noted.[98]

Explanations

The experiences of mental health personnel during the Second World War thoroughly transformed the thrust of psychiatric explanations for traumatic conditions. At the beginning of the war, about two-thirds of American psychiatrists worked in mental hospitals, using biological accounts and somatic treatments for mental illnesses.[99] A much smaller, although influential, psychoanalytical segment of the profession, despite Freud's wartime revisions of his earlier views, focused on early childhood and family influences as determinants of adult mental health. Studies of psychiatric casualties during the war, however, showed that constitutional dispositions, heredity, or personality traits did not predict wartime breakdowns. Instead, by far the most important explanation for which soldiers became psychic casualties was the intensity and duration of their combat experiences.[100]

Psychiatrists came to stress how psychiatrically impaired soldiers responded normally to an abnormal environment. Psychiatrists Roy Grinker and John Spiegel's observation was emblematic:
"It would seem to be a more rational question to ask why the
soldier does *not* succumb to anxiety rather than why he does."[101]
The question shifted from explaining what kind of soldiers would
break down to asking how long it would take for the average soldier to break down. Sociologist Gilbert Beebe and psychiatrist
John Apple calculated that the answer was about eighty-eight days
of constant combat.[102] According to American military psychiatrists Roy Swank and Walter Marchand, "One thing alone seems
to be certain: Practically all infantry soldiers suffer from a neurotic reaction eventually if they are subjected to the stress of modern combat continuously and long enough." Indeed, Swank and
Marchand considered as "aggressive psychopathic personalities"
the less than 2 percent of soldiers who could withstand combat
for an inordinate length of time.[103] The official American report
on the war, *Combat Exhaustion*, indicated that almost all soldiers
broke down psychically after three or four months of incessant
combat. It concluded that "each moment of combat imposes a
strain so great that men will break down in direct relation to the
intensity and duration of their exposure . . . psychiatric casualties
are as inevitable as gunshot and shrapnel wounds in warfare."[104]

The very high rates of psychiatric casualties led to an abrupt
shift in thinking about what factors led to mental disturbance.
During the war, most American psychiatrists underwent a marked
change of view, switching from their initial belief that "a clear cut
distinction [could] be made among men as between the 'weak'
and the 'strong,' to the view that 'every man has his breaking
point.'"[105] By the end of the war, the environmental view that
wartime traumas led *normal* men to develop psychiatric conditions
had prevailed. Explanations involving hereditary dispositions or
neurotic personalities to account for psychiatric casualties almost
completely disappeared. Likewise, earlier suspicions of cowardice
dissipated among military psychiatrists: Grinker's observation that
malingering "is extremely uncommon in this war" was representa-

tive.[106] Instead, researchers focused on factors related to the social organization of military service—on levels of group cohesion, adequate training, and morale—to explain the varying number of psychic casualties across different units. The take-away message was that, when faced with enough environmental stress, all men were likely to break down psychically.

Treatment

At the beginning of the war, military psychiatrists seemed to have forgotten the lessons of World War I regarding the effectiveness of brief periods of rest and relaxation followed by a quick return to the front. Instead, most used treatments involving drugs, hypnosis, and suggestion. Forty-five thousand copies of psychiatrists Roy Grinker and John Spiegel's *War Neuroses*, the "Bible of every new military psychiatrist," were distributed to servicemen.[107] Initially, Grinker and Spiegel assumed that drug-facilitated remembering, along with brief directive psychotherapy, could transform traumatic experiences into healthy memories.[108] They thought that sodium pentothal, in particular, was extremely effective in facilitating the recall of battlefield experiences and thus preventing traumas from becoming ingrained. Other psychiatrists, however, rejected these drugs because they often made users confused and unable to engage in psychotherapy.[109]

Over the course of the war, the emphasis on drug treatments waned while the focus on short periods of rest and relaxation before returning to combat—the treatment of choice by the end of World War I—reemerged.[110] Psychiatrists rediscovered the "PIE principles": treatment should be *proximate* to fighting units rather than removed from the battlefield; *immediate*, so that little time passed between the identification and treatment of a psychiatric casualty; and psychically wounded soldiers should be *expected* to return to combat after a brief period of supportive treatment. Therapies involved simple forms of reassurance combined with rest, sleep, and hot food near the front lines. "Successful treatment," one psychiatrist in the European theater observed, "seemed to depend less on specific procedures or specific drugs than upon general principles—promptness in providing rest and firm emotional support in a setting in which the bonds of comradeship with one's outfit were not wholly disrupted."[111]

Military psychiatrists expected that, when treated appropriately, the vast majority of cases of combat neuroses would be short-lived. William Menninger, the chief of the US Army's Neuropsychiatry Division, claimed that between 30 and 40 percent of neurotic casualties returned to duty within forty-eight hours, and an additional 40 percent recovered within days or weeks.[112] Evaluations of treatment outcomes nevertheless showed mixed results. Some practitioners who used PIE principles claimed to have great success, asserting that about 60 percent of mentally wounded soldiers returned to active duty within two to five days.[113] Other American studies, however, indicated that few soldiers returned to actual combat after treatment.[114] In Britain, too, military physicians conducted research that showed high rates of recovery and return to service. Many of these studies, however, were conducted by the same doctors who treated the soldiers they examined and who thus had a vested interest in showing high recovery rates. The results of studies conducted by more disinterested researchers showed far lower, and highly disappointing, results, of around 10 percent of personnel returned to combat duty.[115]

In contrast to military psychiatrists in the First World War, their counterparts during the second held nearly uniformly sympathetic attitudes toward psychiatric casualties. Their commanders, however, displayed far more mixed responses. Many officers continued to believe that mentally damaged soldiers were cowards or malingerers and to resist therapeutic treatments for combat neuroses. In 1943 the army chief of staff, General George C. Marshall, issued a report claiming that the pain of neurotic soldiers was "nonexistent." Marshall asserted:

> He wears the clothes of an invalid. His food is brought to him. He is catered to by "gray ladies," and, above all, he escapes from those duties which he seeks to evade. He cannot be punished for malingering; therefore, the worst that can happen is to be sent

back to his organization where he can and will start the same process all over again. In the meantime he enjoys a life of leisure with one great goal ahead: to wit, a discharge for physical disability, a comparatively highly paid job as a civilian, a discharge bonus, and eventually a pension from the Veterans Administration Bureau.[116]

Other commanders, however, resisted Marshall's hard line. In 1943 General Omar Bradley issued an order that psychiatric casualties should be seen as cases of exhaustion, "which helped to put to rest the idea that only those men who were mentally weak, 'the unmanly men', collapsed under stress in combat."[117]

Ultimately, Bradley's position prevailed over Marshall's. The most famous incident regarding mental disturbance during the war involved General George Patton. After two hospitalized soldiers told Patton that they were psychiatric casualties, Patton slapped them across the face and called them cowards. By this time (1943), however, conceptions of the legitimacy of psychic breakdowns had changed to the extent that Patton was relieved of his command. This incident is telling, not so much because Patton considered these soldiers to be cowards as because he was punished for his behavior. It was no longer acceptable for officers to disparage the motives of soldiers who psychologically collapsed in combat. Military policy during World War II had come to encourage soldiers to understand and empathize with their mentally disturbed comrades.

Postwar Developments

Psychiatrists and social scientists expected that veterans would face serious problems of social readjustment when they returned home after the Second World War. Sociologist Willard Waller (1899–1945) was the central figure focusing on the social aspects of responses to trauma among returning veterans. "It is clear that the readjustment of the psychoneurotic is fully as much a social as a medical problem," Waller wrote, "and the social aspects of the problem have been neglected."[118] His 1944 book, *The Veteran*

Comes Back, used the readjustment problems of World War I veterans as the model for what he expected soldiers returning from World War II would face when they became civilians. He emphasized that in cases in which relocation to civilian life was easy, the veteran "usually recovers rapidly."[119] But many ex-servicemen would have major difficulties in accommodating to civilian life.

Waller viewed the veteran as "a sort of immigrant in his native land."[120] Many of his problems stemmed from the dramatic differences between military and civilian life. In the army, "nothing counts but women, liquor, and fighting."[121] Conversely, the ideals of duty, loyalty, and bravery, which are paramount for soldiers, are unnecessary in civilian life. Veterans, especially younger soldiers who had no trade to return to, developed deep feelings of resentment because their economic status was lower than that of those who had not fought. They also returned to communities that had been disorganized through migration, housing shortages, and imbalanced sex ratios. These social dislocations meant that the great majority of veterans were acutely estranged for a time before they adjusted to habits of civilian living.[122] Many also faced difficulties of accommodating to the drastic changes in gender roles that had occurred as women on the home front became more self-sufficient. Sharp role reversals emerged as psychically damaged men lost their dominance at home: wives who were formerly dependent on their husbands now became the caretakers of afflicted veterans. "Unless and until he can be renaturalized into his native land, the veteran is a threat to society," Waller warned.[123]

In line with Waller's expectations, many discharged soldiers returned with psychic damage. By 1947 nearly half a million veterans were getting pensions from the Veterans Administration for psychiatric disabilities.[124] These conditions accounted for about 60 percent of all VA patients.[125] But, unlike the period following the First World War (and the American Civil War), no disability crisis arose. A culture of victory prevailed in the United States, which was untouched by the massive destruction of the war. A number of powerful veterans' groups, including the Veterans of Foreign Wars, the American Legion, and the Disabled American

Veterans, successfully lobbied for the GI Bill of Rights. This bill provided rich educational benefits, mortgage assistance, and other forms of compensation for all veterans. The economic prosperity, low unemployment, and growing wealth of the United States in the postwar period insured that pensions for psychiatrically disabled veterans did not overwhelm federal financial resources. The favorable postwar socioeconomic climate made reintegration far more viable than it had been in the aftermath of World War I. Plentiful jobs and high marriage rates among returning servicemen allowed them to integrate into postwar society.[126] "As a consequence there was no place for the experience of trauma of American ex-soldiers," historian Hans Pols concludes.[127]

Postwar culture also focused on issues of social reintegration rather than on psychic disintegration. *The Best Years of Our Lives*, which won the Academy Award for Best Picture of 1947, exemplified this emphasis. It portrayed three veterans who faced difficult transitions into their homes, families, marriages, and jobs: Homer comes home with hooks for hands; Fred has trouble getting work and has an uncaring wife, whom he had married in a shotgun wedding at the outset of the war; and Al is a banker who returns to a wife and children who have established lives of their own. These men occasionally have disturbing memories of combat, but these do not disrupt their lives, and their importance pales before their difficulties of social readjustment.

Traditional conceptions of masculinity, which emphasized stoicism, resilience, and the repression of feelings, prevailed during the postwar period. J. D. Salinger's character Babe, in his short story "Last Day of the Last Furlough" (1944), captures the mood of World War II combatants when he vows that he will never speak about the war once it is over: "I believe . . . that it's the moral duty of all the men who have fought and will fight in this war to keep our mouths shut, once it's over, never again to mention it in any way." Psychiatrists urged wives and families to get vets to talk about their problematic memories of the war and then forget them.[128]

Sloan Wilson's 1955 novel, *The Man in the Gray Flannel Suit*, is the emblematic fictional portrayal of the postwar avoidance of traumatic experiences. Its protagonist, Tom Roth, had many harrowing wartime experiences, including killing one of his own men with a grenade. And yet, "He had not thought of Karkow (Pacific Island) for years."

> The fact that he had been too quick to throw a hand grenade and had killed Mahoney, the fact that some young sailors had wanted skulls for souvenirs, and the fact that a few hundred men had lost their lives to take the island of Karkow—all these facts were simply incomprehensible and had to be forgotten. That, he had decided, was the final truth of the war, and he had greeted it with relief, greeted it eagerly, the simple fact that it was incomprehensible and had to be forgotten. Things just happen, he had decided; they happen and they happen again, and anybody who tries to make sense out of it goes out of his mind.

Tom theorizes about the role of memory: "The past is something best forgotten; only in theory is it the father of the present. . . . The past is gone, Tom thought, and I will not brood about it. I've got to be tough. . . . This is a time of peace and I will forget about the war." He notes, "They ought to begin wars with a course in basic training and end them with a course in basic forgetting." His wife, however, holds a different point of view. "I wish he would talk to me about the war, but I should know better than to try to make him."[129]

Tom Brokaw, the author of *The Greatest Generation*, summarizes the prevailing attitude: "Those of you who returned with unshakable nightmares of war were held through long nights by your uncomplaining wives, and when daybreak came you went off together to resume your lives without whining or whimpering."[130] Unsurprisingly, interest in war neuroses faded in the postwar period.

CONCLUSION

Views of traumatic disorders changed markedly after the beginning of World War I, when traumas were associated with personal vulnerability and emotional weakness. By the end of World War

II, psychiatrists had discarded hereditarian perspectives and assumed that external, contemporaneous shocks were the primary causes of psychic traumas. Everyone, not just a predisposed minority, and men as well as women, was susceptible to traumatic exposure. Nevertheless, medical personnel expected that traumatic symptoms would not last if they were treated immediately, although they granted that some already vulnerable individuals might develop chronic conditions.

The response to PTSD during and after the two world wars shows some distinct differences. Perhaps the starkest divergence was the alteration in symptom presentations across the twenty-five-year period. The classic symptoms of hysteria that emerged among World War I shell-shocked soldiers virtually disappeared in the following war. Instead, symptoms of combat fatigue or combat neuroses during World War II more closely resembled depressive and anxious conditions. The aftermath of the two wars also displayed sharp distinctions in social attitudes toward rewards for disabling psychic symptoms. The strong social resistance to compensating psychologically debilitated veterans of World War I largely evaporated after World War II. Postwar prosperity in the United States both limited the number of veterans who applied for pensions and also facilitated far more compassionate attitudes toward this group.

Explanations for traumatic breakdowns also diverged during the wars. While psychiatrists in both wars debated the relative importance of external events vis-à-vis individual predispositions as primary causes of traumas, over the course of the Second World War the overwhelming weight of opinion turned toward the former. Indeed, conceptions of individual susceptibility to traumas were marginalized within American psychiatry for decades following this war.

The treatment of traumatic psychic conditions across the wars showed both similarities and differences. Responses to psychically traumatized soldiers in World War I were highly varied. Depending on a soldier's particular unit, he might be treated or punished; if treated, he might get drugs, electricity, or psychotherapy and might be referred to a battlefield hospital and quickly returned to combat or be removed to an inpatient facility far from the battle. In contrast, more uniform responses, which focused on the PIE principles, dominated the second half of World War II. The sorts of short-term, rapid, and supportive interventions that were developed during the First World War were assumed to be the best ways to minimize impairments and prevent the formation of chronic symptoms during the Second World War.

The explosion of psychic traumas that emerged from the bloody period of the world wars profoundly shaped mental health policy during the following decades. The dramatic social and economic changes that the New Deal had already brought to American life and thought paved the way for a new environmental emphasis in the culture at large. They legitimated the concept of the welfare state, enlarged the scope of federal intervention in making social reforms, and strengthened the role of psychiatrists in formulating national mental health policies. World War II reinforced the association of highly stressful conditions with massive numbers of mental casualties and anticipated the social emphasis that came to dominate American psychiatry during the 1950s and 1960s. The ideological climate of the postwar period was conducive to sympathetic attitudes toward psychological injuries and the idea that traumatic environments could produce disturbances in otherwise normal individuals.

More than anything else, experiences during World War II led to the belief that environmental stress contributed to mental maladjustment and that purposeful human interventions could alter psychological outcomes. A major reorientation concerning traumatic mental illnesses began, one that emphasized how stress-related mental disturbances were unlikely to become chronic if they received rapid therapeutic responses. Issues of predisposition and malingering receded into the background of mainstream psychiatric thinking during and after the war. Military psychiatrists assumed prominent positions in the government and academia and shaped an environmentally oriented psychiatry that would have major influences on American life in subsequent decades.

CHAPTER FOUR

Diagnosing PTSD

I started flashing back; I was in the Nam; I burned a village
to the ground and everyone in it. I need help.

Eric T. Dean Jr., *Shook over Hell*

By the early 1980s the image of the traumatized, psychologically
impaired veteran had almost totally displaced the image of the
politically active, anti-war veteran in the American memory.

Jerry Lembcke, *Spitting Image*

World War II led psychiatrists to pay far more attention than they
had previously to the relationship between the environment and
psychic maladjustments. In the 1950s and 1960s, psychiatrists revised their understanding of mental illness; they now believed that
social stressors, more than the qualities of predisposed individuals,
were responsible for the bulk of mental disturbances. The most
influential American psychiatrist during the immediate postwar
period, William C. Menninger, concluded that the "history or the
personality make-up or the internal psychodynamic stresses" were
less important than "the force of factors in the environment which
supported or disrupted the individual."[1] In addition, the wartime

focus on brief, immediate treatments that took place near combat units strongly impacted postwar government policies, which emphasized community mental health.

Modeled on the tenets of military psychiatry, sweeping changes in attitudes and responses to mentally ill persons marked the postwar period. Mental health became a widespread social concern and a pressing national problem. A psychosocial model that viewed social conditions as a primary cause of psychological problems prevailed. The basic concept behind the idea of war neuroses—that environmental stressors led to psychic breakdowns—was applied to a wide range of conditions. Family and socioeconomic pathologies as well as intra-individual disturbances came to be viewed as the cause of many psychological disorders.[2] This understanding profoundly influenced public policy toward mental illness.

During the 1950s and 1960s, as the federal government encouraged the development of community treatment facilities, mental institutions began to empty. This community-oriented model assumed that early treatment interventions with people who had mild maladjusted states could prevent more severe conditions from developing.[3] Robert Felix, the first director of the National Institute of Mental Health (NIMH), observed how "the impact of the social environment on the life history, and the relevance of the life history to mental illness[,] are no longer serious questions as clinical and research findings"—that is, social environment and life history had been established as causes of mental illness.[4] The NIMH funded many projects that sought the roots of mental disturbances in environmental sources, including poverty, racism, and family interactions.

Major changes in the relationship between gender roles and mental health also began in the 1960s and escalated in the following decades. Males traditionally resisted expressing emotion and vulnerability and so were unlikely to seek mental health treatment, which signaled their failure as men. Military culture, in particular, emphasized toughness, stoicism, and the ability to resist fear. The rise of feminism challenged this traditional conception of masculinity. The growth of the women's movement was especially congruent with the emergence of a therapeutic culture that underscored the need for both sexes to openly display their emotions and admit their vulnerabilities. The current post-traumatic stress disorder diagnosis was formulated within this rapidly changing cultural climate.

DSM-I AND DSM-II

Before World War II psychiatric classifications gave short shrift to traumatic neuroses. Emil Kraepelin's canonic work in the late nineteenth and early twentieth centuries did mention "fright neurosis," a category that encompassed railway spine, but it was marginal to his nosology. The only reference to trauma in the predecessor to the *DSM-I*, *The Statistical Manual for the Use of Hospitals for Mental Diseases*, which guided psychiatric classification in the United States between its first edition in 1918 through its 10th edition in 1942, was a category of "psychoses due to trauma." This category was restricted to psychotic reactions that "were brought about by head or brain injury as a result of force directly or indirectly applied to the head."[5] Yet, such psychotic reactions were rarely found among combatants, who were far more likely to display symptoms of traumatic neuroses.

After World War II a consensus arose about two aspects of traumatic conditions. First, external factors were a central cause of mental illness. In 1946, Menninger advocated for a "renewed appreciation of the importance of stress from social forces as a major factor in the causation of psychiatric casualties."[6] Second, although combat neuroses were very common, they were likely to be transient unless predisposing factors were present.[7] Men who entered military service without vulnerabilities to neuroses were unlikely to develop persistent psychopathologies during and after combat. During and soon after the war, Menninger developed a new psychiatric nomenclature for the army that reflected these assumptions.[8] It focused on the sorts of acute combat states, stress responses, and personality disturbances that combatants displayed.

The manual located combat experiences under the new category of "transient personality reactions to acute or special stress."[9]

Menninger's taxonomy became the basis for the *Diagnostic and Statistical Manual of Mental Disorders* (*DSM-I*), which was published in 1952. The wartime experiences of military psychiatrists inspired the creation of the manual. Following the prevailing psychosocial tenets at the time, the *DSM-I* focused on the underlying personality dynamics and external causes of the various conditions it described, paying scant attention to their symptoms. Historian Gerald Grob describes it as reflecting "the intellectual, cultural, and social forces that had transformed psychiatry during and after World War II."[10]

The *DSM-I* divided mental disorders into two major groups. The first encompassed those conditions in which impaired brain functioning led to mental disturbances. In a nod to the original conception of shell shock, this group included categories of "Acute Brain Syndrome associated with trauma" and "Chronic Brain Syndrome associated with brain trauma," which produced lasting impairments of mental function.[11]

The manual emphasized the second group, which included the sorts of condition that were rarely found among the hospitalized patients the earlier *Statistical Classification* had featured: "Only about 10% of the total cases seen [during the war] fell into any of the categories ordinarily seen in public mental hospitals."[12] The *DSM-I* was highly attuned to conditions that arose from external stress: "The 'psychoneurotic label' had to be applied to men reacting briefly with neurotic symptoms to considerable stress; individuals who . . . were not ordinarily psychoneurotic in the usual meaning of the term."[13] It included the vast majority of cases resembling war neuroses within the category "Transient situational personality disorders," under the subcategory "Gross stress reaction." This diagnosis stated: "Under conditions of great or unusual stress, a normal personality may utilize established patterns of reaction to deal with overwhelming fear. The patterns of such reactions differ from those of neurosis or psychosis chiefly with respect to clinical history, reversibility of reaction, and its transient character. When promptly and adequately treated, the condition may clear rapidly. . . . The particular stress involved will be specified as (1) combat or (2) civilian catastrophe."[14] Gross stress reactions were both reversible and transient.

Following the lead of World War II military psychiatrists, who assumed that "every man has his breaking point," the criteria clearly indicated that most trauma victims were "normal people" who found themselves in abnormal situations: "In many instances this diagnosis applies to previously more or less 'normal' persons who have experienced intolerable stress." Also in line with wartime experiences, these conditions were not expected to endure: "When promptly and adequately treated, the condition may clear rapidly." In contrast, chronic states that resulted from trauma were more likely to be due to some other condition: "If the reaction persists, the term is to be regarded as a temporary diagnosis to be used only until a more definitive diagnosis is established."[15] In other words, the traumatic stress that previously normal people experienced will generally be temporary and self-healing or responsive to brief treatments. The manual did not entertain the idea that traumatic stress, in itself, would produce chronic symptoms among people who lacked some preexisting vulnerability.

During the period between the publication of the *DSM-I* in 1952 and 1968, when the manual entered its second edition (*DSM-II*), the postwar influences of military psychiatrists waned. No organized group retained an interest in trauma-related diagnoses. Although the *DSM-II* kept a diagnosis of "Psychosis with brain trauma" that developed immediately after a severe head injury, it dropped the category of gross stress reaction. It replaced it with a general diagnosis of "Transient situational disturbances," which was "reserved for more or less transient disorders of any severity (including those of psychotic proportions) that occur in individuals without any apparent underlying mental disorders and that represent an acute reaction to overwhelming environmental stress."[16] As in the first *DSM*, this condition was expected to be short-lived: "If, however, the symptoms persist after the stress is

removed, the diagnosis of another mental disorder is indicated."
The nomenclature also contained a subcategory of "Adjustment
reaction of adult life" and used as one of three examples "Fear associated with military combat and manifested by trembling, run-
ning and hiding"—virtually the definition of cowardice.[17] Neither
of the first two DSMs, therefore, incorporated any diagnosis in
which an environmental stressor led to persistent symptoms. The
absence of any category that encompassed chronic or long-delayed
combat-related stress became highly significant when psychologically disturbed veterans returned from the Vietnam War.

VIETNAM

The Vietnam War featured combat situations thoroughly unlike
those in previous conflicts. A large conventional American force
faced small guerrilla bands that attacked unexpectedly. Battle lines
rarely existed, and most encounters with the enemy involved surprise attacks, usually at night. Combatants were also confronted
with various hidden improvised explosive devices, mines, and
booby traps, which caused many casualties. Civilians, including
women and children, were often indistinguishable from enemy
soldiers.

Few American soldiers found that the war had any meaningful
purpose, their major goal was to stay alive. The average age of US
soldiers in Vietnam was just nineteen years, compared to the mean
age of twenty-six years during World War II. Heroin and other
powerful drugs were widely available and helped these soldiers
deal with the stress of the war. Unlike in previous wars, troops
were not rotated in and out as units; instead, each individual spent
a defined term of service. The individual rotation system "priva-
tized the war experience and encouraged [soldiers] to function as
separate individuals," according to sociologist Paul Starr.[18]

The number of psychological casualties during the Vietnam
War itself was strikingly low, just 12 per 1,000, considerably fewer
than the 37 per 1,000 in the Korean War, and ten times less than in
World War II.[19] They accounted for less than 5 percent of all military evacuees.[20] The prevailing view at the time was that mental

health practices in Vietnam had been a resounding success. The military attributed the small number of mentally disturbed personnel chiefly to the policy of establishing immediate treatment responses by embedding psychiatrists in frontline combat units. "Psychiatric casualties," Peter Bourne, the head of the army's Psychiatric Research Team, observed in 1970, "need never again become a major cause of attrition in the United States military in a combat zone."[21]

The initial studies of returning Vietnam veterans failed to find widespread psychic impacts of combat: one major report indicated that 7 percent of veterans had a full depressive syndrome, a rate that was not much higher than in the general population.[22] Another examination of about 600 veterans and nonveteran controls found that the nearly 25 percent of veterans it classified as maladjusted did not exceed the rate among nonveteran controls.[23] Remarkably, the very high rates of heroin use among soldiers in Vietnam sharply declined to minimal levels once "addicted" veterans had returned home.[24] Paul Starr's research showed that, contrary to stereotypes, Vietnam veterans were no more violent than others of comparable social backgrounds.[25] The issue of suicide was also prominent at the time, but, again, studies showed rates no higher among veterans than among same-aged men in the general population.[26] Most veterans adjusted well in objective terms: they had higher median incomes than and similar unemployment rates as their peers. Moreover, Vietnam veterans who were in combat earned higher incomes than noncombatants.[27]

Despite low rates of trauma-related mental conditions during the war and of generally good patterns of readjustment after it, prevailing cultural images of Vietnam veterans depicted troubled men who were prone to violence, suicide, and mental disturbance. Many media portrayals of veterans featured characters who had become crazed by their wartime experiences. In stark contrast to the cinematic portrayals of heroic and self-sacrificing World War II soldiers, popular films such as *Taxi Driver*, *Deer Hunter*, and *Coming Home* featured suicidal and homicidal veterans. Others focused on the pointlessness of the war and the atrocities that

American forces had committed. For example, a veteran on one television show stated: "I started flashing back; I was in the Nam; I burned a village to the ground and everyone in it . . . I need help."[28] Movies that depicted flashbacks among veterans were particularly potent vehicles for showing how past wartime traumas could intrude into the present: when triggers arose in their current environments, subjects vividly reexperienced the original shock.[29] One film critic complained, "So familiar has this story become that I have started to think of it as a brand new film genre—the PTSD (Post-Traumatic Stress Disorder) genre."[30]

Images of widespread pathology among Vietnam veterans were widely accepted because they symbolized the pervasive cultural and political rifts that split the country at the time. The postwar society the veterans had entered was riven by deep divisions and lacked the social cohesion that marked American society after World War II and the Korean War. Veterans' problems became entangled with the moral revulsion that many people felt toward the war. The "Vietnam veteran serves as a psychological crucible of the entire country's doubts and misgivings about the war," historian Eric Dean observed.[31]

Deep controversy still exists about the responses that returning Vietnam veterans received. One common conception is that they were treated like outcasts by a society that scorned their wartime service. In this account, even older veterans at the American Legion and VFW posts derided those returning from Vietnam.[32] Psychiatrist Nancy Andreasen's assertion is representative: Vietnam veterans "returned home to find that (unlike previous generations of soldiers) they were not warmly welcomed as heroes, but instead sometimes vilified as social pariahs."[33] Others, however, claim that veterans were warmly welcomed when they returned.[34] They cite polls taken at the time indicating that almost all veterans thought they had a "friendly" reception when they arrived home, and they regarded the supposed humiliations suffered by Vietnam veterans, such as being spat upon, as unwarranted urban legends.[35] Sociologist Jerry Lembcke contends: "I not only found no evidence that anyone was ever spat on, but no evidence either that anyone at the time said he had been spat on."[36] Neverthe-less, "the image of the Vietnam veteran as a spurned, neglected, and troubled individual has refused to die."[37] Whatever the true story, the prevailing assumption that veterans were traumatized, scorned, and humiliated came to shape the development of the PTSD diagnosis.

ANTIWAR PSYCHIATRY

An influential advocacy group, Vietnam Veterans Against the War (VVAW) emerged in the late 1960s. It thoroughly contrasted with veterans' groups in previous conflicts. The VVAW did not focus on obtaining pensions and other compensatory resources, which had been the chief goal of veterans' advocacy efforts after past wars; instead, it fervently opposed the war itself, the government that was conducting the war, and the Veterans Administration (VA), which it insisted was neglecting veterans' problems.[38] In particular, the VVAW emphasized what it asserted were routine atrocities committed by American troops against the Vietnam-ese. This claim became the basis for a powerful narrative about the psychic impact of Vietnam on combatants: the psychological problems that veterans faced resulted from governmental policies that forced them to participate in or witness war crimes.[39] A new conception of soldiers as traumatized victims of an unjust war emerged. Although the VVAW only involved a small proportion of veterans, it was well-organized, attuned to the media, and allied with prominent psychiatrists.

The VVAW emerged in a cultural climate that emphasized the political dimension of psychiatric diagnoses. During the 1960s, prominent critics of psychiatry such as Thomas Szasz, R. D. Laing, and Erving Goffman focused on how labels of mental illness were political tools used to enforce conformity. The problems mental illness created did not so much stem from afflicted individuals as from a deformed social order and a repressive psychiatric profes-sion. Psychiatrists working with Vietnam veterans reshaped this focus to show how diagnoses could also serve political ends that *benefited* their recipients. In contrast to the antipsychiatry critics, the VVAW desired psychiatric labels that drew attention to their problems.

Although there was no extant recognized diagnosis that served the purposes of veterans' advocates, the experiences of Holocaust survivors in many ways provided a model of the psychic costs of traumas. One highly relevant aspect of the Holocaust for Vietnam veterans was that Jews and other victims who survived the concentration camps were not screened or selected but indiscriminately exposed to appalling conditions. More than any other traumatic circumstance, the long-term psychiatric impacts of the camps were due to a horrific situation, not to any individual characteristics. The question to be explained was not which survivors became mentally ill but instead which few were able to successfully adapt to such extreme circumstances.[40]

A second contribution that the Holocaust literature made to the veterans' view of trauma was to render irrelevant issues of malingering, cowardice, and secondary gains from psychic injuries that had been central to previous discussions of stress-related diagnoses. There was no question that survivors of the extermination camps had undergone horrendous experiences. In addition, veterans adopted the notion of survivor guilt, which had initially emerged in psychoanalyst Bruno Bettelheim's writings about Dachau and Buchenwald, as a characteristic symptom of traumatic conditions.[41] Victims felt guilty because so many of their fellow combatants had perished while they had survived.

Another influential impact of the Holocaust was to provide support for the veterans' contention that traumatic psychological symptoms were not transient but could be prolonged or delayed. This feature was especially important because it contradicted the assumptions of stress-related diagnoses before the *DSM-III*, which had emphasized how persistent symptoms were due to individual predispositions rather than traumatic events.

Equally important, post-Holocaust accounts provided a new model of the professional-client relationship for mental health professionals working with Vietnam veterans.[42] Psychoanalysts like the American William Niederland, who coined the phrase "survivor syndrome," did not view their role as embodying dispassionate observation. Instead, they actively joined the efforts of wronged victims who sought reparations for their psychic injuries from German courts.[43] Just as the experiences of Holocaust survivors provided a template for the commonality of trauma victims, the activist responses of their clinicians showed that psychiatrists and other mental health professionals should not be passive purveyors of therapy.

Beginning in the early 1970s, the VVAW established therapeutic groups, which they called "rap groups," modeled after the consciousness-raising sessions of the women's movement. These self-organized sessions took place outside of established psychiatric clinics and of the US Department of Veterans Affairs (VA), which the veterans scorned.[44] In them, participants talked about their feelings regarding wartime experiences.[45] Discussions focused on veterans' estrangement, mistrust, and anger toward the American military and government.

The conceptions of masculinity that the VVAW promoted diverged markedly from ones in previous eras. It rejected traditional male values of pride of service, fondness for battle, fearlessness in the face of danger, and expertise in killing.[46] Instead, rap groups encouraged members to display their soft and defenseless qualities and to reveal feelings to others.[47] They emphasized the vulnerability and sensitivity of combatants who suffered from the brutality they were forced to inflict on civilians and soldiers. A psychiatrist allied with the VVAW summarized: "They grappled with alternative modes of maleness put forth by youth culture: being gentle, open, non-competitive, 'soft' (to the point of being able to cry), aesthetically sensitive . . . responsive to the needs and struggles of individual women."[48]

The VVAW had an outsized influence over portrayals of traumatic mental illnesses in the 1970s. One of its allies, psychiatrist Chaim Shatan, coined the term "post-Vietnam syndrome" in a widely read 1972 op-ed piece in the *New York Times*.[49] This syndrome emerged from the experiences that veterans recounted in rap groups. It was inseparable from the VVAW's intensely moral, antiwar sentiments. The post-Vietnam syndrome featured themes of atonement, scapegoating, and "hatred of Orientals," which were far afield from traditional psychiatric diagnostic criteria.

Psychiatrist and political crusader Robert Jay Lifton (1926–) was the most influential psychiatrist affiliated with the VVAW. A prominent critic of the war, Lifton scorned military psychiatrists, comparing them to Nazi doctors in concentration camps who collaborated with an "absurd and evil organization," the US military.[50] Lifton's earlier work on the Japanese survivors of the bombing of Hiroshima had focused on the concept of survivor guilt, which Lifton then applied to Vietnam veterans. His notion of PTSD differed from prior conceptions because he believed that wartime stressors were not necessarily traumatic at the time they occurred. They only became highly disturbing at a *later* date, when veterans realized how morally repugnant their actions had been. The indelible images that haunted veterans are "always associated with guilt," he claimed.[51]

Lifton's primary goal was to use the psychological damage to veterans as a reason for ending the war. His book *Home from the War* (1973) focused on the disturbed veterans who participated in the VVAW rap groups. It emphasized the moral aspects of war-related traumas among Vietnam veterans, many of whom had committed atrocities and suffered from a deep sense of survivor's guilt. They could only be cured, Lifton stressed, after admitting that they were war criminals. Under the conditions of the Vietnam War, "moral revulsion and psychological conflict became virtually inseparable, sometimes in the form of delayed reactions."[52]

Home from the War was enormously successful and became a major influence on media portrayals of returned veterans. Only a few critics objected to Lifton's depictions. One was Paul Starr, who claimed that Lifton had created the psychiatric problems he claimed he had found among veterans. In fact, Starr asserted, survivor guilt was rarely found among veterans but instead was "very prevalent among those who write about Vietnam veterans."[53] The

VVAW, Starr emphasized, was a small and unrepresentative group that did not provide an accurate reflection of the psychic problems veterans faced.

While most veterans associated with the VVAW scorned the VA, some VA personnel became their dedicated allies. The patients of VA social worker Sarah Haley, a well-known advocate of the VVAW, became the most celebrated examples of traumatized veterans. Haley claimed that on her first day of work at a VA hospital she was approached by a terrified veteran who was diagnosed with paranoid schizophrenia. This man stated that he had been threatened with death if he revealed a massacre he had seen in Vietnam. When Haley recounted his story at a staff meeting she was "laughed out of the room."[54] In 1974 Haley wrote a widely cited article in the *Archives of General Psychiatry* that described the conditions of 130 VA patients. Haley emphasized the differences between the mental disturbances of these Vietnam veterans and those of veterans of previous wars. She focused on the 40 patients who said they had committed war crimes. Many were so traumatized by their actions that they had repressed the most painful details of their atrocities. Haley asserted that "many veterans did not react immediately to this stress and only became 'psychiatric casualties' months and even years after their return to the United States."[55] Such delayed reactions to their atrocities typified the veterans she treated.

Lifton, Shatan, and Haley were the most influential of many highly politicized mental health professionals who were active adversaries of the military and who strove to undermine the government's pursuit of the war. They became notable voices in the media, which broadcast their claims that widespread pathology existed among returning veterans, that many vets had committed atrocities, and that enormous numbers were addicted to drugs or had attempted suicide. These clinicians deemphasized traditional forms of treatment and urged therapists to identify with their patients and veterans and to become involved in political protests against the war.[56]

The hostility to the Vietnam War also penetrated deeply into the American Psychiatric Association (APA). In 1970 its Board of Trustees passed a statement: "The board hereby expresses its conviction that the prompt halt to the hostilities in Southeast Asia and the prompt withdrawal of American forces will render it possible to reorder our national priorities to build a mentally healthy nation."[57] Two years later, the organization further asserted: "We find it morally repugnant for any government to exact such heavy costs in human suffering for the sake of abstract concepts of national pride or honor."[58]

The construction of the PTSD diagnosis was thus intrinsically connected to the political and moral turmoil surrounding the war. A group of politically committed veterans, psychiatrists, and their allies at the VA were driven by the idea that an immoral war had done serious psychological damage to its participants. In addition, they were outraged that the governmental bodies most concerned with the plight of veterans, the US Congress and the Veterans Administration, resisted giving any special consideration to their psychological problems.[59] Historian Edgar Jones and psychiatrist Simon Wessely observe that the origins of the PTSD diagnosis lie "less in the jungles of Vietnam and more in the socio-political climate of America in the Vietnam era."[60]

The VVAW and allied psychiatrists became the leaders in political lobbying and media appeals for a diagnosis that would provide veterans with treatment, compensation, and reparations for their service.[61] Yet, because few had been diagnosed with war-related conditions during their periods of active service and because so much time had passed since the initial trauma occurred, they did not fit the criteria for any extant *DSM-II* diagnosis. They required a new condition, whose symptoms were not just products of some environmental stressor but could also emerge or persist many years after the trauma that had provoked them.

DSM-III

The agitation of the VVAW and its professional allies during the 1970s occurred during a period when the classification system of psychiatric diagnoses was undergoing a dramatic reconfiguration.

In 1974 the APA appointed Robert Spitzer to head a task force charged with revising the *DSM-II*. Spitzer led a small, but powerful, group of research-oriented psychiatrists whose work required carefully defined conditions that would not vary across different sites. This group was devoted to the idea that psychiatry must become a legitimate branch of medicine. At the core of medical thinking was the notion of disease specificity. Historian Charles Rosenberg explains: "This modern history of diagnosis is inextricably related to disease specificity, to the notion that diseases can and should be thought of as entities existing outside the unique manifestations of illness in particular men and women: during the past century especially, diagnosis, prognosis, and treatment have been linked ever more tightly to specific, agreed-upon disease categories."[62] Spitzer anticipated that all diagnoses in the new manual would adhere to the principle that they were true diseases, which could be identified without reference to the lived experiences of those who suffered from them. This standard stood in stark opposition to the veterans' belief that their personal wartime involvements were intrinsic aspects of their subsequent psychic conditions.

Spitzer and his allies sought to create a reliable diagnostic system—one in which different psychiatrists who saw the same patient would agree on what condition they observed. They believed that only careful distinctions between the manifest symptoms of different disorders could produce such a classification. Specific, empirically derived, and reliable criteria must be the basis for each psychiatric diagnosis. Therefore, definitions of all conditions would feature explicit and detailed lists of their accompanying symptoms. In addition, each diagnostic entity would be distinct from other diagnoses. The *DSM-III* would be based on empirical observation, not theoretical speculation, and on science, not clinical intuition. These core principles stood in thoroughgoing opposition to the unconscious mechanisms, general psychosocial stressors, and overlapping conditions that the analytically oriented *DSM-II* had relied on.[63]

Spitzer also strove to eliminate the psychodynamic causal attributions that marked the extant diagnostic manual because he believed that the causes of mental disorders were not yet known. A potential PTSD diagnosis contradicted the principle that diagnoses would be a-causal because, by definition, PTSD was linked to some trauma. Above all, the new system had to be based on purely medical criteria: it could not encompass the moralistic concerns that had marked the post-Vietnam syndrome. The proponents of a new PTSD diagnosis, therefore, had a very rough road to travel before they could insert a traumatic condition into the new, medically minded manual.

Advocates pushed for a diagnosis that would recognize traumatic symptoms as a normal response to an immoral war, absolve veterans from blame, and allow them to receive treatment and compensation. To this end, they asserted that post-traumatic stress disorder had to be grounded in thoroughly environmental causes with no role for individual predispositions: they "argued that the only significant predisposition for catastrophic stress disorders was the traumatic event itself."[64] The Holocaust provided them with a paradigmatic situation of a trauma whose impact would produce dire consequences, regardless of individual factors. Equally important, because the most intense period of the Vietnam War had ended more than ten years before the *DSM-III* was published in 1980, advocates required a diagnosis that recognized that traumatic symptoms could persist for many years beyond the initial trauma or could emerge well past the time the trauma had occurred.

If the causal thrust of a diagnosis that acknowledged that traumatic events could produce psychic impacts in otherwise normal people was inconsistent with the assumptions of the *DSM-III* Task Force, it accorded with a central line of psychiatric thinking over the previous hundred years. From Erichsen and other proponents of railway spine, to Freud's later work, to the views of Kardiner and the World War II psychiatrists, and finally to the general principles behind psychiatric classifications from William Menninger through the *DSM-I* and *DSM-II*, external traumas were assumed to play a major role in why some people developed mental disturbances. Moreover, the focus on how stressors caused psychic disorders was highly compatible with the cultural climate of the 1960s and 1970s, which emphasized how social factors produced mental illness.

Despite the congruence of the stressor basis of traumatic conditions with one strand of psychiatric history, the advocates for a PTSD diagnosis had a number of hurdles to overcome. One was that a stressor-based diagnosis was not consistent with the militantly a-causal paradigm that Spitzer and his allies promoted as the model for the *DSM-III*. Not surprisingly, they initially resisted a PTSD category because it intrinsically involved a causal framework. In addition, allies of Spitzer who had studied traumatic conditions argued that there was no need for the new manual to include a *distinctive* PTSD diagnosis. In particular, prominent epidemiologist Lee Robins claimed that the existing categories of depressive and anxiety disorders could incorporate most veterans' symptoms.[65] Indeed, one study found that less than 2 percent of patients had PTSD conditions that were not accompanied by some other psychiatric diagnosis.[66] Robins and others believed that a particular category of PTSD was superfluous as well as unsupported by empirical research.

Another obstacle that advocates faced was that *DSM-III* diagnoses required specific lists of symptoms that would serve as definitional criteria. The broad aspects of PTSD-like conditions were well-recognized since at least the time of Freud's later work.[67] The previous literature on traumatic conditions, however, was relatively unconcerned with constructing the detailed symptomatic measures that the *DSM-III* demanded; instead, it contained a large and multifaceted array of psychic consequences of traumas. Past work also focused on the general impact of traumas on emotional and social functioning rather than on their particular symptoms.

An additional problem was that the most influential past observers of traumatic conditions thought that these conditions were unlikely to be enduring in the absence of predisposing factors.

This association of individual susceptibilities with chronicity was not acceptable to the advocates of a new diagnosis, who required a focus on external stressors for persistent or long-delayed as well as for acute conditions. "After such massive man-made stress," Shatan emphasized, "preexisting disorder is irrelevant. The specific stress itself constitutes the crucial predisposition."[68]

Moreover, the antiwar psychiatrists had to contend with the prior consensus that most combat conditions would respond to short periods of rest and relaxation and that few would become chronic unless symptoms led to secondary gains. For example, Kardiner devoted a lengthy section of his book to compensation, which he saw as the major factor that would block recovery. For him, the promise of monetary rewards for veterans did not create traumatic illnesses but it did impede their successful treatment and rehabilitation: "Once the patient learns that his disability can be used as a means of compelling the world to recognize his claims for dependency, it is then often too late to begin treatment with any chance of a successful issue."[69] Recovery would also lead to the loss of compensation, which gave patients a powerful incentive to remain ill. The idea that veterans would use their symptoms to obtain secondary gains was completely alien to the antiwar psychiatrists, who resisted any suggestion that enduring PTSD symptoms were anything other than genuine.

Despite the considerable impediments they faced, Lifton and Shatan were able to persuade Spitzer to appoint them and a Vietnam veteran, Jack Smith (the sole member of the roughly 150 persons on the various *DSM* task forces to have no graduate degree), to the six-member advisory committee working on the Reactive Disorders section of the new manual. Spitzer named Nancy Andreasen, a prominent psychiatrist at the University of Iowa, as chair of the Reactive Disorders Task Force. Andreasen had studied the psychiatric complications associated with severely burned adults.[70] Her work focused on the anxiety, depression, regression to infantile states, and occasionally, delirium that burn victims suffered. The veterans' advocates realized that they would have to convince at least one additional member (the others were psychiatrist Lyman Wynne and Spitzer himself) to secure a diagnosis that could displace blame from the soldier onto the war itself.[71]

In contrast to the other major diagnoses in the *DSM-III*, no specific research was conducted on the PTSD criteria before the diagnosis entered the manual. It had none of the trappings of other conditions—no field trials, tests of reliability, or statistical analyses of data. Researchers had not compared different criteria sets to select the best alternatives. Instead, the driving force behind the diagnosis was the political agitation of antiwar psychiatrists and veterans' advocates who relied on the moral argument that failing to include a PTSD diagnosis in the new manual would be tantamount to blaming victims for their misfortunes.[72] In an ideological climate that was still highly charged from the aftermath of the war, their moral position transcended the data-driven arguments that prevailed in the creation of other diagnoses. Sociologist Wilbur Scott concluded that PTSD is in *DSM-III* "because a core of psychiatrists and veterans worked consciously and deliberately for years to put it there. They ultimately succeeded because they were better organized, more politically active, and enjoyed more lucky breaks than their opposition."[73]

PTSD IN THE DSM-III

The post-traumatic stress disorder diagnosis that emerged in the *DSM-III* (see table) had three fundamental components: its definition of a traumatic stressor, the particular symptoms that were likely results of the stressor, and the division of acute and chronic traumas. The stressor criterion required the "existence of a recognizable stressor that would evoke significant symptoms of distress in almost everyone."[74] It thus fully embraced veterans' concern over displacing any responsibility for symptoms from the environment to the individual. The text accompanying the diagnostic criteria only mentioned the issue of possible predisposing factors in passing: "Preexisting psychopathology apparently predisposes to the development of the disorder."[75] It specified that qualifying traumas are "outside the range of usual human experience," en-

DSM-III Diagnostic Criteria for Post-traumatic Stress Disorder

A. Existence of a recognizable stressor that would evoke significant symptoms of distress in almost everyone.

B. Reexperiencing of the trauma as evidenced by at least one of the following:
(1) recurrent and intrusive recollections of the event
(2) recurrent dreams of the event
(3) sudden acting or feeling as if the traumatic event were reoccurring, because of an association with an environmental or ideational stimulus

C. Numbing of responsiveness to or reduced involvement with the external world, beginning sometime after the trauma, as shown by at least one of the following:
(1) markedly diminished interest in one or more significant activities
(2) feeling of detachment or estrangement from others
(3) constricted affect

D. At least two of the following symptoms that were not present before the trauma:
(1) hyperalertness or exaggerated startle response
(2) sleep disturbance
(3) guilt about surviving when others have not or about behavior required for survival
(4) memory impairment or trouble concentrating
(5) avoidance of activities that arouse recollection of the traumatic event
(6) intensification of symptoms by exposure to events that symbolize or resemble the traumatic event

Source: American Psychiatric Association, Diagnostic and Statistical Manual of Mental Disorders, 3rd ed. (Washington, DC: American Psychiatric Association, 1980), 238.

compassing severe stressors such as military combat, rape, assault, and natural or man-made disasters.[76] The PTSD diagnosis therefore provided a unifying framework for all kinds of severe traumas, giving "legitimacy to the fact that victims of rape, assault, military combat, airplane crashes, fires, floods, bombing and torture can suffer psychological trauma with symptoms that are debilitating and life changing and that should not be denied."[77]

The symptom criteria for the diagnosis required, first, that the trauma be reexperienced through intrusive recollections, recurrent dreams, or feelings of reoccurrence. Second, sufferers had to show numbed responsiveness through diminished interest in activities, detachment from others, or constricted affect. Finally, they had to display at least two symptoms from among hyperalertness, sleep disturbance, survivor guilt, trouble concentrating, avoidance of reminders of the traumatic event, and intensification of symptoms following such reminders.[78]

The third component of the diagnosis was this: "Symptoms may begin immediately or soon after the trauma. It is not unusual, however, for the symptoms to emerge after a latency period of months or years following the trauma."[79] Acute PTSD involved symptoms that arose within six months of the trauma and disappeared within this time frame. Chronic PTSD either persisted for longer than six months or arose sometime after six months had passed since the trauma. This aspect of PTSD responded to veterans' need for a diagnosis that recognized that symptoms need not arise during or soon after a wartime trauma but might only become apparent at a much later date.

PROGENITORS OF THE PTSD DIAGNOSIS

The PTSD diagnosis that emerged in the *DSM-III* in 1980 to recognize the suffering of Vietnam veterans was a thoroughgoing paradigm shift in the conceptualization of psychiatric trauma. In contrast to previous notions of shell shock or combat neuroses, which were expected to be acute and self-healing unless the affected soldier had some predisposing condition, PTSD was thoroughly environmental. Contrary to previous conceptualizations, the idea of individual vulnerabilities had no role in the new conception. Like previous diagnoses, it arose from some external cause, but unlike its predecessors, this cause worked through present-day *memories* of the past trauma that intruded into the present. What were the intellectual predecessors of these diagnostic criteria?

Abram Kardiner's book *The Traumatic Neuroses of War*, based on the World War I veterans he had treated during the 1920s (although the book was not published until 1941), was an especially influential precursor of the stressor criteria.[80] According to Ben

Shephard, "Ultimately, Kardiner would prove the most influential writer on the war neuroses. In the 1970s, when American medicine was confronted by an epidemic of mental disorders in Vietnam veterans, his book was a bible, almost the only thing the psychiatrist could turn to."[81] Yet, Kardiner's thought itself was an outgrowth of Freud's wartime conception that traumatic neurosis arose as "a consequence of an extensive breach being made in the protective shield against stimuli."[82] Kardiner, following Freud, considered traumas to be situations in which sudden, external stressors overwhelmed the capacity of individuals to deal with the stimulus: "*Trauma*, therefore, is an *external* factor which initiates an abrupt change in previous adaptation."[83] Although he treated traumatized male soldiers, Kardiner believed that wartime neuroses did not differ in any fundamental way from other traumas, except that they are usually more intense.[84] Therefore, it was easy for the PTSD working group to extend his conception to natural disasters, rape victimization, and other extreme traumas.

Kardiner's rejection of both biological and psychological susceptibilities for traumatic neuroses also appealed to the antiwar psychiatrists. Kardiner found that sufferers from these conditions had every possible type of preexisting personality, and he concluded that predispositions could not be important causes. "If therefore we look for the predisposing factors in the pre-traumatic personality we are not likely to find anything distinctive," Kardiner stated.[85] Instead, following Freud's revised conception, he emphasized the importance of viewing symptoms as adaptations that were attempts to gain mastery over traumatic situations. The stressor criterion was also in tune with the environmental emphasis of post–World War II psychiatry and culture, if not with the *DSM-III*'s a-causal approach.

The origins of the PTSD symptom criteria are more obscure. Chaim Shatan claims that he, along with Jack Smith and Sarah Haley, were "practically dictating" the text of the diagnostic criteria to Nancy Andreasen.[86] Aside from the mention of survivor guilt as partially fulfilling the "D" requirement, however, the symptoms that found their way into the manual were not present in Shatan's previous, highly moralistic, work. Andreasen herself asserts that she was the primary author of the text, although the symptom criteria involving intrusive recollections, numbing, and hyperalertness, which are the most prominent features of the *DSM-III* diagnosis, for the most part did not appear in her publications about the burn victims she had studied.[87]

In one of the great ironies of psychiatric history, the PTSD symptom criteria most closely resemble Sigmund Freud's wartime views. Spitzer and the other research psychiatrists behind the *DSM-III* were contemptuous of psychoanalytic approaches. Nevertheless, the B criteria of "recurrent and intrusive recollections of the event; recurrent dreams of the event; and sudden acting or feeling as if the traumatic event were reoccurring" almost completely mirror Freud's view of trauma that emerged from World War I.[88] In contrast, Kardiner's portrayal of symptoms, which had more in common with the hysterical presentations soldiers displayed during and after World War I, had little resemblance to the PTSD symptoms. His concept of physioneuroses focused more on the general bodily and personality processes that traumas acted upon than on their particular symptoms.[89]

The numbed responsiveness found in the C criteria and potpourri of symptoms in the D criteria closely resemble psychiatrist Mardi Horowitz's work. His research investigated responses to traumas through experimental studies using films about stress, fieldwork that looked at symptom formation after a variety of stressors, and clinical investigations of patients after dire events. These studies were particularly important because they contained the type of empirical findings that the *DSM-III* Task Force valued most highly. This research, along with Horowitz's 1970 book *Image Formation and Cognition*, emphasized the phasic alteration between intrusion and avoidance.[90] It focused on how traumatized people often relived vivid images of traumatic events that were not subject to their control, and yet at other times they were unable to remember the trauma. Horowitz's well-known book *Stress Response Syndromes* was published in 1976 (it has undergone three subsequent revisions), while the deliberations for the *DSM-III* were under way. The book developed a cohesive portrayal of the stress syndrome, which involved a "constellation of denial, repression, and emotional avoidance" that was strongly influenced by Freud's later views.[91] Most of the symptoms in the *DSM-III* criteria are found in Horowitz's compilation of common stress responses, which focused on the paradoxical and seemingly contrasting symptoms of repetition and denial.[92]

The third component of the PTSD diagnosis that gives equal weight to acute and chronic conditions also relied on Horowitz's work. Previous psychiatrists, including Freud and Kardiner, believed that most traumatic symptoms would be short-lived. Freud doubted the lingering impact of war trauma: "When war conditions ceased to operate, the greater number of the neurotic disturbances brought about by the war simultaneously vanished."[93] Kardiner, too, wrote: "These traumatic neuroses do not get worse with time; I have never seen a case that was worse at the time I saw it, than at any time previous."[94]

In contrast, Horowitz's work featured chronic as well as acute forms of PTSD. Horowitz emphasized how a minority of people who have acute cases will develop persisting symptoms or develop symptoms after a period of latency.[95] He noted how the very low rate of psychiatric casualties during the Vietnam War itself did not preclude the emergence of genuine disorders well after the war had ended. In the postwar period, "the denial and numbing, the alienation, compartmentalization, and isolation of the experience from everyday life would continue for a while. Paradoxically, it might only be with the vision of continued safety, with the permissible relaxation of defensive and coping operations, that the person might then enter a phase in which intrusive recollections of the experience were reemergent."[96] After a latency period of apparent relief, full-scale stress syndromes, including nightmares, intrusive images, and emotional attacks related to the wartime experiences, could emerge.

The new diagnosis reoriented responses to PTSD. The *DSM-III* criteria were perfectly suited to the needs of antiwar veterans and their advocates. Because it was unequivocally environmental

in orientation, the role of possible biological or psychological predispositions almost completely disappeared. Traumas caused, not
just triggered, symptoms. PTSD diagnoses thus allowed veterans
to see themselves as victims of an unjust war, a conception that
was in tune with the antiwar cultural climate that still prevailed.
It also rendered veterans eligible to receive disability payments and
psychiatric treatment. At the same time, it contained the detailed,
explicit list of symptoms that the new classificatory system required. It also fit the requirement that previously unscathed people could develop PTSD many years after the trauma had ended.
The antiwar veterans and psychiatrists, in tandem with the PTSD
Work Group, overcame the *DSM-III* Task Force's general antipathy to causally based diagnoses.

THE IMPACT OF THE PTSD DIAGNOSIS

The extent of post-traumatic stress disorder after the Vietnam
War was a highly charged and controversial topic. Studies had
found that veterans of World War II and Korea did not have worse
mental health later in life compared to civilians.[97] Indeed, when
surveyed in 1996, more than 90 percent reported that their mental
health was "good to excellent" compared to 84 percent of nonvet-
erans. Another study of more than 400 male veterans of World
War II and Korea conducted in 1990 found that less than 1 percent
of veterans had a current PTSD diagnosis and that just 1.5 percent
met diagnostic criteria at some point in their lives.[98] A survey of
152 World War II veterans who were assessed for symptoms in
1946 and of a subset of 107 surviving veterans in 1988 found that
only one met *DSM-III* diagnostic criteria for PTSD.[99] Psychiatrist
George Vaillant's prospective study of 268 Harvard graduates, 152
of whom served in World War II, uncovered only one full-blown
and four partial cases of PTSD.[100] Other retrospective studies
indicated that World War II veterans rarely developed delayed
PTSD. A representative national survey found that these veterans
had better mental health in later life than those who hadn't served
in the military.[101]

The initial studies of PTSD among Vietnam veterans found

similarly low rates. The most prominent was the Centers for Disease Control's large Vietnam Experience Study (VES). It found that only 2 percent of veterans had PTSD at the time the study was conducted, although 15 percent met diagnostic criteria at some point during the war. "Vietnam veterans seem to be functioning socially and economically in a manner similar to army veterans who did not serve in Vietnam," the study concluded.[102]

Subsequent to 1980 interest also grew in the prevalence of PTSD in the general population, not just among combatants, who had been the focus of prior work. Studies of communities using the *DSM-III* criteria found quite low rates of PTSD. The initial research was part of the Epidemiologic Catchment Area (ECA) research, a pioneering study of mental disorders in five US regions conducted shortly after the *DSM-III* was published, in 1980. Using the initial *DSM-III* measures, which required the presence of extraordinary stressors, it found modest rates of the disorder. Data from the St. Louis site found that only 5 men and 13 women per 1,000 met PTSD criteria at any time during their lives. Indeed, only Vietnam veterans who had been wounded in combat reported high levels of PTSD. The overall prevalence was just 1 percent.[103] Another study using data from the North Carolina ECA site found a similarly low 1.3 percent lifetime prevalence and a six-month prevalence of just 0.44 percent.[104] PTSD, as defined by the *DSM-III* criteria, rarely occurred in the general population. While the *DSM-III* provided the groundwork for the subsequent surge of PTSD, changes to the diagnostic criteria in future manuals, far more than the *DSM-III* itself, resulted in the dramatic growth in traumatic conditions that arose in the 1990s and that continues to the present.

CONCLUSION

The PTSD diagnosis that emerged in the *DSM-III*, in contrast to the other diagnoses in the manual, maintained the focus on environmental causes of mental disorders that had been within the mainstream of psychiatric thought since World War II. It also contained the specific list of symptoms that was necessary for any psychiatric condition to be considered a true medical disorder. The diagnosis thus allowed sufferers to receive treatment, compensation, and substantiation of their conditions. It validated new conceptions of masculinity, which recognized that men as well as women were vulnerable to the psychic consequences of traumas. Finally, PTSD legitimated the view that traumas could have lasting consequences as well as have a period of latency, so symptoms might not appear until many years after the original trauma. The clinical community consensually agreed that the new condition was a positive development.[105] Only a few gadflies questioned whether it might produce large numbers of chronic sufferers who would otherwise have displayed natural self-healing of their traumas.[106]

Despite the research in the aftermath of the *DSM-III* that indicated quite low rates of post-traumatic stress disorder, the notion that PTSD was pervasive spread through the general culture. The PTSD diagnosis quickly shaped portrayals of traumatic conditions: "By the early 1980s the image of the traumatized, psychologically impaired veteran had almost totally displaced the image of the politically active, anti-war veteran in the American memory."[107] A new age of trauma had begun.

CHAPTER FIVE

The Return of the Repressed

The most common post-traumatic disorders are those not
of men in war but of women in civilian life.

Judith Herman, *Trauma and Recovery*

In but a few years we will all look back and be dumbfounded by
the gullibility of the public in the late twentieth century and by
the power of psychiatric assertions to dissolve common sense.

Paul McHugh, Foreword to August Piper Jr., *Hoax and Reality*

Women's traumas had been at the heart of psychiatric attention
before the First World War. Between that war and the establishment of the post-traumatic stress disorder diagnosis in the *DSM-
III*, wartime traumas that afflicted men took center stage in discussions about stressor-related conditions, but then, during the
interlude between 1980 and the Persian Gulf War in the 1990s,
concern with veterans' mental health problems faded. Although
feminist clinicians had little involvement in creating the PTSD
criteria, once the diagnosis appeared they saw its relevance to their
concerns: traumatized females who were victims of male violence
and abuse. At this time, the central focus of attention to traumas

turned from the ravages of combat to the lasting consequences of childhood sexual abuse.

The psychological devastation of traumas that men inflicted on women became a significant theme within one branch of feminism. In the 1980s a backlash developed against the theme of sexual liberation, which had been prominent in feminist efforts during the 1960s and 1970s—decades when the women's movement emphasized the rights of women to have the same sexual freedoms as men, reproductive choice, and equality in work and family roles. In the eighties, many leading feminists, including Catherine McKinnon, Andrea Dworkin, and Gloria Steinem, vocally expressed their concerns that the sexual freedom of recent years had produced even more male oppression over women than previously.[1] They focused on the sexual exploitation of women by men, emphasizing the dire impacts of family violence, date rape, workplace sexual harassment, and childhood sexual abuse. "Perhaps incestuous rape," Dworkin proclaimed, "is becoming a central paradigm for intercourse in our time."[2]

In the 1980s, too, a seeming epidemic of male violence against women broke out. Many feminists trumpeted the findings of sociologist and activist Diana Russell's survey in San Francisco, which found that one in four women had been raped and one in three abused in childhood.[3] Russell claimed that over 25 percent of her respondents were victims of sexual abuse before the age of fourteen and 12 percent were incest victims. Prominent feminist psychiatrist Judith Herman proclaimed, "Father-daughter incest is not only the type of incest most frequently reported but also represents a paradigm of female sexual victimization."[4]

Along with reports of rising rates of sexually abused women, women suddenly began to report recovering memories of forgotten incidents of sexual abuse, often incestuous, during their childhood. They rarely recalled isolated traumas but instead recollected repeated occurrences that had taken place over long periods. Most of them only remembered these events after entering psychotherapy many years later. Some accounts claimed that as many as half of American women had suffered repressed incidents of childhood sexual abuse.[5] Even the lowest estimates regarded 1.6 million American girls and women as incest victims.[6] The elicitation of repressed sexual abuse in childhood grew "from virtual nonexistence to epidemic frequency."[7]

Recollection of prolonged and repeated childhood traumas became common among psychiatric patients: "On careful questioning, 50–60 percent of psychiatric inpatients and 40–60 percent of outpatients report childhood histories of physical or sexual abuse or both," Herman concluded.[8] One of the leaders of the recovered memory movement, psychologist Renee Frederickson, summarized: "Finally, I realized the size of the problem. Millions of people have blocked out frightening episodes of abuse, years of their life, or their entire childhood. They want desperately to find out what happened to them, and they need the tools to do so."[9]

As a result, a stark change in the gendered relevance of traumatic mental illnesses occurred in the 1980s. The women's movement realized, according to Herman (perhaps the most prominent psychiatric theorist of women's trauma), that "the most common post-traumatic disorders are those not of men in war but of women in civilian life."[10] The stereotypical image of a trauma victim changed from a battle scarred veteran to a woman who was psychically incapacitated from childhood sexual abuse.

THE RECOVERED MEMORY MOVEMENT

The recovered memory movement (RMM), which swept the United States in the 1980s, focused on the lasting, albeit unconscious, impacts of childhood traumas. It comprised a coalition of patients, mostly middle- and working-class white women (over 90 percent of cases were women), activist mental health professionals, and lay promoters.[11] Leading psychiatrists such as Herman and Bessel van der Kolk at Harvard and Lenore Terr at the University of California–San Francisco provided the professional authority for the movement.[12] They were joined by a large group of non-MD and often noncredentialed psychotherapists who actively encouraged the recovery of repressed memories of early sexual traumas. Like the Vietnam Veterans Against the War (VVAW) and its associated mental health professionals, advocates associated with the RMM saw their mission as a moral crusade, in this case against patriarchal violence. They viewed fathers as the most common perpetrators of repressed traumas involving sexual abuse. Like the crusading associated with the situation of Vietnam veterans, mental health professionals associated with the RMM felt they had a moral obligation to be passionate advocates for their clients, not just neutral interpreters of symptoms. The mass media widely appropriated their tenets and promoted recovered memories as a source of popular entertainment and potential imitation.

Mental health personnel involved in the recovered memory movement asserted that, in contrast to typical cases of PTSD, in which past traumatic events are vividly remembered, traumatic conditions associated with early sexual traumas were so powerful that they left no conscious trace in memory. Instead, they were precisely, if unconsciously, encoded in the brain, awaiting their recovery in psychotherapy. The process of "robust repression"— memories of severe abuse that remained in a pristine state within the unconscious until they were uncovered later in life—was at the core of women's traumatic conditions.[13] Although the events that repressed memories referred to occurred many years before they were recovered, patients could come to remember their early traumas in perfect detail. Echoing Freud, historian Alison Winter suggested that recovered memories were like the discovery of an old record that had never been played.[14]

Historical Origins

The historical roots of the recovered memory movement were far removed from the wartime experiences that influenced the *DSM-III* PTSD diagnosis. Instead, the surge in interest about psychopathologies related to recovered memories of childhood sexual abuse revived the late nineteenth-century concerns of Pierre Janet and, far more ambivalently, of Sigmund Freud.

Freud's unwavering assertions that childhood sexual secrets lay behind the later formation of neurotic symptoms was a foundational claim for the recovered memory movement. Indeed, Freud anticipated almost every one of its tenets.[15] Nevertheless, recovered memory theorists and clinicians were typically hostile, often aggressively so, toward Freud's writings. One of the leaders of the movement, psychiatrist Colin Ross, indicated: "Freud did to the unconscious mind, with his theories, what New York City does to the ocean with its garbage."[16] Gloria Steinem went even further, proclaiming that "sending a woman to a Freudian therapist . . . is not so far distant from sending a Jew to a Nazi."[17]

Freud's original formulation was that all cases of hysteria stemmed from "one or more occurrences of premature sexual experience, occurrences which belong to the earliest years of childhood but which can be reproduced through the work of psycho-analysis."[18] Within a year, however, he changed his view that patients suffered from repressed memories of actual sexual abuse to the notion that they repressed their own erotic attractions to parents of the opposite sex. The sexual abuse that analysts uncovered did not involve real incidents but instead represented patients' unconscious fantasies.

A major reason for Freud's repudiation of his initial seduction theory was that hysteria was widespread in late nineteenth-century Vienna. If every hysterical case resulted from sexual abuse, as Freud asserted, then adults were exploiting young children and even infants at an astonishing rate. According to Richard von Krafft-Ebing, who, as the foremost student of sexual pathology at the time was hardly unfamiliar with childhood molestation, Freud's view seemed "like a scientific fairytale."[19] Freud also changed his original assertion that governesses, family friends, older siblings, and strangers seduced his patients when they were children, instead declaring that their fathers were the source of patient-remembered abuse. Freud's revised theory was of cold comfort to RMM advocates because these paternal seductions were nothing more than imagined products of repressed desires.

Recovered memory advocates accepted Freud's initial claims but scorned his revised view regarding the fantasies behind childhood traumas. The same assertion about the huge prevalence of early sexual abuse that had led Viennese psychiatrists to reject Freud's initial claims was exactly what appealed to the RMM. One of their central contentions was that sexual abuse of female children by adult males, especially fathers, was extensive. Those associated with the RMM harshly criticized Freud's repudiation of his original view and avowed that patients suffered from genuine sexual victimizations. Psychiatrist Jeffrey Masson's attack on Freud's abandonment of the seduction theory in his best-selling 1984 book, *The Assault on Truth: Freud's Suppression of the Seduction Theory*, was especially influential.[20] Masson avowed that Freud had betrayed the victims of severe abuse because he feared the reactions of his male colleagues, who strove to uphold the patriarchal authority that dominated Viennese culture. Freud knowingly protected the pedophile fathers of his patients, whom he sacrificed to protect male privilege, while relegating patient abuse to the influence of unconscious fantasies. Subsequently, to its detriment, psychoanalysis became the study of fantasy and desire, not of lived experiences.

Herman and others revived Freud's original, self-repudiated seduction theory, arguing that repressed memories of sexual abuse, often incestuous abuse, caused traumatic symptoms. She declared that Freud's initial paper was "a brilliant, compassionate, eloquently argued, closely reasoned document."[21] Herman insisted that Freud's patients recovered memories of real sexual assault, abuse, and incest. In contrast, Freud's revised theory led to the situation in which "the dominant psychological theory of the next century was founded in the denial of women's reality."[22]

As an alternative to Freud, a number of the founders of the recovered memory movement, including Herman and van der Kolk, resurrected the generally forgotten writings of Pierre Janet, Freud's contemporary and sometime rival.[23] Traumas had been at the core of Janet's writings and clinical practice. Recovered memory advocates were especially attracted to his concept of dissociation. Janet developed the idea that the psychic impacts of traumas were so powerful that they could not be integrated into the personality.

This led traumatized victims to develop a form of consciousness that was inaccessible to their awareness. Their memories remained intact, if unconscious, in this dissociated state, although therapists might be able to recover them through techniques such as hypnosis. This notion of storing memories of traumas in an unconscious region of the mind was at the core of the recovered memory movement. "Instead of remembering being what affected us," philosopher Ian Hacking summarized, "it was the forgetting."[24]

However useful Janet's emphasis on dissociation was for the recovered memory movement, unlike Freud, Janet did not focus on sexual traumas but instead often described sicknesses, accidents, deaths of relatives, and other unpleasant experiences as the origin of dissociated states. The RMM was less interested in the types of traumas that Janet discussed and treated than in his focus on how the natural psychological defense against traumas was for the mind to protect itself by blocking memories of the abuse while retaining them in a hidden part of the psyche.

The recovered memory movement also revived the interest in split personalities that had arisen in France at the end of the nineteenth century. Janet and other late nineteenth-century French psychologists and psychiatrists (including Charcot) had discussed a few cases of multiple personality disorder (MPD), a condition in which several distinct personalities were present within the same individual. Psychiatrist Morton Prince (1854–1929) led a movement to publicize this condition in the United States. Most MPD patients at the time typically displayed a small number of distinct personalities. The condition, however, was uncommon. "This phenomenon is, upon the whole, rather rare, and it is unlikely you will have to occupy yourselves with it in practice," Janet told an audience at Harvard Medical School in 1908.[25] By 1944, MPD had virtually disappeared; in that year a comprehensive survey uncovered only seventy-six cases in the medical literature over the previous 128 years.[26] Another survey uncovered only fourteen cases between 1944 and 1969, half of which were patients of one psychiatrist, Cornelia Wilbur.[27] Accordingly, psychiatric manuals before the *DSM-III* did not mention MPD.

After a considerable period of latency, MPD cases began to emerge and spread through American popular culture. Two best-selling books (both made into popular movies)—the *Three Faces of Eve* (1957) and *Sybil* (1973)—provided prototypes for this condition. In 1973 Wilbur published the famous case of Sybil, which became a staple of reading lists in undergraduate psychology courses. Sybil, in contrast to her French predecessors, had a large number of alter egos, ranging into the teens. According to Wilbur and a colleague, "MPD is most parsimoniously understood as a post-traumatic dissociative disorder of childhood onset."[28] Her promotion of this condition would lead many women to emulate Sybil's condition. By 1990 over 20,000 cases had been diagnosed in the United States.[29]

The Tenets of the Recovered Memory Movement

The recovered memory movement reincarnated and amplified the major concerns of European psychiatry during the 1890s. Like Janet and Freud, proponents of recovered memories focused on the lasting, if unconscious, impacts of childhood traumas. Their core assumption was that memories of abuse remained in a pristine state within the unconscious until they were uncovered later in life. Another key tenet of the RMM was that the childhood traumas bringing women to therapy were often not isolated events. Instead, they were more likely to involve long periods of repeated traumas so painful that victims could not incorporate them into consciousness. They were thus most likely to repress prolonged episodes of early sexual abuse. Herman proposed that a syndrome of "complex post-traumatic stress disorder," which encompassed the results of continuous and repeated abuse, best captured the nature of traumas associated with recovered memories. She invoked the prolonged symptoms of the survivors of the Nazi death camps, as well as studies of soldiers during World War II, to emphasize the psychic persistence of long-standing traumas. Like these groups, victims of patriarchal abuse suffered repeated instances of abuse but could not flee from their oppressors.[30]

A third notable aspect of the RMM, comparable to the Vietnam veterans' advocacy during the 1970s, was the central role that nonprofessionals played in both groups. By the early 1980s, the rise of third-party insurance and managed care, the new centrality of biological views, and the prominence of drug treatments had marginalized psychoanalysts within the psychiatric profession. At the same time, the PTSD and MPD diagnoses discussed below opened a new landscape of traumas that could be treated and re-imbursed. Numerous non-MD counselors, psychologists, social workers, and uncredentialed psychotherapists filled this vacuum. Most of these clinicians were women, many of whom held ex-plicitly feminist views of therapy.[31] The advocacy efforts of the VVAW and its psychiatric allies provided feminist clinicians with an example of the power of political and moral activism to influ-ence mental health policy and practice.

Some of the movement's basic texts emerged from lay survivors of early abuse. In particular, poet Ellen Bass and short-story writer Laura Davis's *The Courage to Heal*, published in 1988, became a canonical work. The authors had no background in psychology but were radical feminists who relied on "the experiences of survi-vors."[32] Their core belief was that sexual abuse during childhood was common and often repressed but that it could be brought to consciousness through the assistance of sympathetic therapists. Between 1988 and 1992 the book sold 750,000 copies and to this day remains a best-selling self-help text.[33]

Bass and Davis strove to reach women who had repressed memories of molestations by showing them the signs that indi-cated the likelihood of earlier traumas. They created checklists that encompassed an extraordinary range of signs of abuse. These included items such as having trouble feeling motivated, having no sense of one's interests, talents, or goals, and feelings of pow-erlessness (among many others), which indicated that the reader was likely to have suffered from repressed childhood traumas. The authors emphasized how accounts of abuse are never false: "So far, no one we've talked to thought she might have been abused, and then later discovered that she hadn't been. The progression always goes the other way, from suspicion to confirmation. If you think you were abused and your life shows the symptoms, then you were."[34] Indeed, Bass and Davis claimed that not one of the hundreds of women they spoke with who suspected that they had been abused turned out to be wrong. Moreover, *not* believing one had been abused could itself be a sign of abuse.

The RMM embraced another tenet of late nineteenth-century psychiatry: to remember is to heal.[35] Sufferers of repressed memories, therefore, must recover and reexperience their early traumas in the present moment. The anguish of earlier traumas could only be overcome when repressed memories were brought to consciousness with the aid of knowledgeable clinicians. Once memories had been recalled, they were relived with vivid accuracy, down to the smallest detail of the original traumatic event.

Following Charcot, Janet, and the early Freud, clinicians frequently used hypnosis as an aid to recovery. For many patients, hypnotic trances provided the most direct and immediate ways of recollecting painful memories that were otherwise inaccessible to experience. Therapists assured patients that under hypnosis they could activate parts of the mind that are usually not available to them.[36] They often supplemented hypnotic sessions with sodium amytal, cocktails of tranquilizers, or antipsychotic drugs. Recovered-memory clinicians assumed that repressed memories that were uncovered through these methods provided accurate portrayals of long-forgotten traumas.

Therapeutic responses expanded beyond the clinical encounter itself as the idea spread that recalling and then discussing traumas within the treatment setting was a necessary, but not a sufficient, aspect of healing. Instead, the notion of giving voice to traumatic memories, which had emerged in studies of Holocaust survivors, spread to feminist therapists. "The conflict between the will to deny horrible events and the will to proclaim them aloud is the central dialectic of psychological trauma," Herman declared.[37] Women who recovered memories of early abuse were encouraged to think of themselves as "survivors," who would give public voice to their traumas and avenge their perpetrators: "These days, in voicing one's own traumas, one assumes a moral authority vis-à-vis the past that trumps questions of both factual truthfulness and practical efficacy. Speaking becomes its own truth," trauma scholar Michael Roth observed.[38]

Harkening back to the era of railroad spine, the recovered memory movement also used lawsuits as a way of gaining recompense from perpetrators. In the case of accusations spawned by recovered memories, however, offenders were not large corporations and their insurers but fathers and other relatives.[39] For feminists, such litigation was less a process to obtain monetary compensation as it was a form of therapy. Bass and Davis stressed how "nearly every client who has undertaken this kind of suit has experienced growth, therapeutic strengthening, and an increased sense of personal power and self-esteem as a result of litigation. Clients also feel a tremendous sense of relief and victory. They get strong by suing."[40] The courts joined the couch as a venue for therapeutic healing.

Concern about obtaining justice for recovered memory victims spread to state legislatures, which passed bills that extended the statute of limitations to forgotten crimes that were only remembered many years or even decades later. The recovered memory movement's assumptions became embedded in legislation that started the clock for when defendants could be held liable for traumatic abuse from the time memories were recovered rather than from the time of the original event.[41] By 1991, twenty-one states had made exceptions to statutes of limitations for recovered memory cases. Victims flooded the courts with cases seeking punishment and compensation from fathers and other caretakers whom they accused of abuse. Like therapists, police and prosecutors did not question stories about forgotten histories of sexual abuse. Law enforcement personnel rarely challenged victims' accusations, even when they involved horrendous crimes, including recovered memories of witnessing killings, dismemberments, and eating babies during sessions of devil worship.[42]

Patients who recovered memories of early traumas required some diagnosis that would pay for their therapy. Their clinicians needed to classify clients within a *DSM* diagnostic category to be compensated for their efforts. PTSD was not a completely satisfactory condition for these purposes.

TRAUMATIC DIAGNOSES

Recovered memory proponents admired the openly moralistic concerns of the veterans and their allies who lobbied for the posttraumatic stress disorder diagnosis. While antiwar and antigovernment concerns propelled veterans' advocacy efforts, feminist politics was the driving force behind the recovered memory movement. Echoing the connection between antiwar psychiatrists and traumatized veterans, Herman wrote, "Early investigators often felt strong personal bonds and political solidarity with trauma survivors, regarding them less as objects of dispassionate curiosity than as collaborators in a shared cause."[43] In both cases, therapists viewed their traumatized patients' problems as political, not just medical. Clinicians must affirm "a position of moral solidarity with the survivor. . . . It is morally impossible to remain neutral in this conflict. The bystander is forced to take sides," Herman maintained.[44]

The central quality of the PTSD diagnosis that emerged in the *DSM-III* in response to the conditions of traumatized veterans also resonated with the advocates of recovered memories of childhood sexual abuse. The symptoms of male veterans and abused women had a common etiology in overwhelming external traumas that produced psychological disturbances. The purely environmental focus of PTSD was highly suited to feminist concerns; trauma victims suffered from outside forces that were beyond their control. Any possible predispositions they might have were secondary to the abuse they suffered.

Yet, the *DSM-III*'s PTSD diagnosis was not entirely apt for the conditions of women who recovered memories of early childhood abuse. All of the stressors that the manual mentioned—combat, disaster, rape, assault, serious accidents, and the like—were relatively contemporaneous with resulting symptoms. Unlike the stressors associated with PTSD, the traumas that female victims came to remember took place when they were children or even infants. While the PTSD diagnosis did allow for delayed onset of symptoms, its criterion of a six-month or longer interval between a trauma and its resulting symptoms was not intended to apply to conditions that only emerged many years, or even decades, after experiences that had begun in early childhood.

Another divergence between the RMM and the PTSD criteria was in their respective views of the relationship between trauma and memory. The central problem for PTSD sufferers was the "recurrent and intrusive" nature of their traumatic memories.[45] In thoroughgoing contrast, the very first sentence of Herman's *Trauma and Recovery*, the RMM's central professional text, stated that "the ordinary response to atrocities is to banish them from consciousness."[46] Victims did not recall these horrendous events until after they had entered therapy. The repression of traumatic experiences had little connection to the intrusive memories of veterans and others, who were tormented by their recollections of traumas.

A third difference between the PTSD diagnosis and the traumas that the RMM featured regarded the psychic conditions that traumas produced. The PTSD criteria were only satisfied if patients reported enough specific symptoms that related their current memories and activities to some past trauma. Mental health professionals allied with the RMM, however, associated daily sexual traumas with a broad range of indicators. These encompassed depression, anxiety, anger, sexual dysfunction, psychosomatic disorders, low self-esteem, loneliness, interpersonal difficulties, and multiple personality disorder, among others.[47] Van der Kolk, in a nod to Kardiner, emphasized how the body, if not the mind, remembers traumas through converting repressed psychological symptoms into numerous physical problems that tyrannized patients by emerging in disguised forms.[48] The critical aspect of recovered memories of childhood traumas was not their particular symptomatic results, which differed widely across patients, but the capacious psychic and bodily impacts of childhood abuse. These distinctions rendered the PTSD criteria less than optimal for the RMM.

By the mid-1980s, the recovered memory movement had become a significant presence among mental health professional and lay therapists. A large cadre of clinicians had arisen who were committed to using techniques that brought memories into consciousness after many years of repression. This group required criteria that recognized that traumatic experiences could be repressed as well as intrusive. The revised criteria of PTSD in the *DSM-III-R* (1986) responded to this aspect of memory by changing the category of numbed responsiveness to the external world to include the "inability to recall an important aspect of the trauma."[49] Traumatic symptoms now encompassed the incapacity to remember some trauma as well as recurrent and intrusive memories of it. This change helped expand the realm of PTSD from male victims of combat and other stressors to sexually abused women who had repressed long-ago traumas. "By the end of the decade, reluctance to disclose became inability to remember," psychologist Richard McNally observed.[50]

Although the revised *DSM-III-R* criteria were more attuned to the RMM than the initial *DSM-III* diagnosis, the psychic conditions found among the victims of early childhood traumas often did not fit the PTSD stipulations. Instead, the RMM became enamored with the long-neglected condition of multiple personality disorder (MPD). Although it was little noticed at the time, the *DSM-III* contained a separate diagnosis for this disorder. The manual briefly described MPD as "the existence within the individual of two or more distinct personalities, each of which is dominant at a particular time" and had "its own unique behavior patterns and social relationships."[51] The distinctive quality of MPD was its florid, overt presentation of a variety of characters who speak in different voices. As with the other *DSM* diagnoses, PTSD notwithstanding, the manual did not specify the causes of MPD, although it noted that child abuse and other severe emotional childhood traumas could be predisposing factors. In line with psychiatric history, the *DSM-III* asserted that "the disorder is apparently extremely rare."[52]

In the first half of the 1980s, MPD became a prominent concern of mental health professionals. Typical patients had never recognized the existence of their many personalities until they entered treatment with a therapist who specialized in treating this condition.[53] By 1986, the first revision of the *DSM-III*, the *DSM-III-R*, observed that "recent reports suggest that this disorder is not nearly so rare as it has commonly been thought to be."[54] In that year, a National Institute of Mental Health psychiatrist estimated that "more cases of MPD have been reported in the last 5 years than in the preceding two centuries."[55] The *DSM-III-R* criteria also implicitly associated MPD with recovered memories, noting that the "onset of Multiple Personality Disorder is almost invariably in childhood, but most cases do not come to clinical attention until much later." In addition, the text said, "Several studies indicate that in nearly all cases, the disorder has been preceded by abuse (often sexual) or another form of severe emotional trauma in childhood."[56] After 1986, the association of MPD with early childhood traumas and repressed memories of sexual abuse made it the diagnosis of choice for many clinicians associated with the RMM.

The changes in the PTSD and MPD diagnoses both responded to and contributed to the flourishing of the recovered memory movement. "Repressed memory became the preeminent psychological topic of the late 1980s, and a defining feature of public debate," historian Alison Winter noted.[57]

THE SPREAD OF THE RECOVERED MEMORY MOVEMENT

The mass media propelled women's traumatic mental illnesses to general public attention.[58] Awareness of forgotten memories of sexual abuse that adults had experienced as children rapidly spread from therapeutic circles to public consciousness. Traumas, especially those related to repressed memories of sexual abuse in early childhood, became a conspicuous aspect of television programming, the publishing industry, and popular culture.

The most celebrated cases associated with the RMM played out not in the confines of therapeutic encounters but before millions of spellbound television viewers or readers of popular publications. The dramatic revelations of recovered memory victims became staples of daytime talk shows, popular magazine stories, self-help books, and survivor therapy groups. Celebrities such as television actress Roseanne Barr discovered and publicly discussed their recovered childhood traumas; a *People* magazine cover story about Barr, "I Am an Incest Survivor," appeared in 1991.[59] Television personalities Phil Donohue, Sally Jessie Raphael, Geraldo Rivera, Larry King, and Oprah Winfrey (who said she was herself a victim of incest as a child) sympathetically portrayed survivors and demonized their abusers. Moreover, they viewed victims not as isolated cases but as exemplars of a large and growing epidemic.

The pervasive media coverage of recovered memories led many women to wonder if they, too, might have repressed traumas involving sexual abuse in their own lives. They then sought confirmation of their suspicions from sympathetic therapists. Typical cases of repressed memories involved adult women who accused their fathers of dreadful crimes, including incestuous rapes, aborting fetuses that were the results of these rapes, and forced sex with animals and groups of men. Recovered memories of ritual abuse by satanic cults, including watching murders and rapes, became another prominent motif.

Perhaps the best-known account was Lawrence Wright's *Remembering Satan: A Tragic Case of Recovered Memory* (1994).[60] Wright related the story of Paul Ingram, a deputy sheriff in Washington State and a member of a charismatic religious movement that emphasized the power of Satan. Ingram confessed to (but later repudiated) accusations of sexual molestation from his daughters, who were twenty-two and eighteen at the time of the charges. Their allegations spread to their mother, brothers, friends of the father, and members of a satanic cult who killed babies, one of whom was aborted from the older daughter. Curiously, both women also claimed to be virgins. Eventually, his daughters accused Ingram of raping one of their brothers as well as themselves, of arranging gang rapes at poker nights with his friends, of forcing them to have sex with dogs and goats, and of having murdered many babies at gatherings of satanic cults. The daughter who made the first allegation had previously read a book describing satanic cults that mutilated and sacrificed babies.

Ingram initially didn't remember anything about any of these charges but soon confessed to having frequent sex with both daughters since the time the oldest was five years old. Later, he remembered police dogs raping his wife, group orgies, satanic rituals, and murdering prostitutes among many other incidents. Sociologist Richard Ofshe was able to get Ingram to confirm a story that Ofshe himself implanted that involved him forcing his daughter to have sex with one of his sons—an outcome that indicated Ingram's extreme suggestibility to whatever charges he was accused of.[61]

Ingram pleaded guilty to six counts of third-degree rape, although at his sentencing hearing he proclaimed that he was not guilty and had never sexually abused his daughters. Wright's book makes clear that a psychologist, a preacher, and detectives who believed the incredible, and constantly shifting, stories that his daughters told had implanted Ingram's recovered memories. They convinced Ingram that most sex offenders did not remember their crimes and suggested that he had lost memories of abuse he had suffered as a child, which he obligingly soon remembered. None of the interrogators questioned any element of the accusers' stories, however implausible they might have been.

In another celebrated case a California woman, Eileen Lipsker, revealed recovered memories of her father, George Franklin, raping and then murdering her friend two decades earlier. Noted psychiatrist Lenore Terr, who later wrote the book *Unchained Memories* about the case, testified that Lipsker had remembered nothing of this event until she recovered it in psychotherapy.[62] Terr emphasized how Lipsker's detailed memories, which she had repressed for twenty years, precisely mirrored the crimes she had witnessed. On the basis of her testimony, despite the lack of any material evidence implicating him in the crime, Franklin was sentenced to life in prison. After revelations that Lipsker's memories were produced under hypnosis and after a number of witnesses retracted their testimony, a higher court reversed his conviction on the grounds that recovered memories were not reliable.[63]

Over the brief course of the RMM movement, attention came to focus on claims of satanic ritual victimization.[64] Such cases became regular television fare, where alleged victims described chilling tales of baby killings, mutilations, forced abortions, and the like. The influential talk show host Geraldo Rivera's "Devil Worship: Exposing Satan's Underground" became one of the most watched documentaries in television history.[65] According to Rivera, "Satanic cults: every hour every day, their ranks are growing. . . . The odds are that this is happening in your town."[66] In 1990 a survey found that about a third of members of the American Psychological Association treated clients who had suffered from such abuse.[67] Nearly all believed that these claims were true. Prominent psychologist D. Corydon Hammond proposed that many such victims of abuse were raised in satanic cults that originated in Europe, with roots in Hitler's SS and extermination squads.[68]

Settings that took care of small children were another locus of traumatic incidents involving satanic cults. Perhaps the best known arose in 1983 concerning the Virginia McMartin Preschool in California. The owner and her son were charged with sexually molesting 360 children in their care over a ten-year period. The initial complainant, the mother of one of the children, asserted that her son described sexual rituals, animal sacrifices, and abductions in airplanes. Later plaintiffs spoke of copulations between naked nuns and priests, having pencils and other objects stuck up anuses and vaginas, and watching horses killed with baseball bats. Within a year allegations of similar abuse had spread to sixty-three other day-care centers in the Los Angeles area alone.[69] In another spectacular trial in 1987, Margaret Kelly Michaels, a day-care worker at Wee Day Care in Maplewood, New Jersey, was convicted of 131 counts of sexual assault–related crimes against preschool children.[70] Michaels served five years in prison before the New Jersey Supreme Court overturned the earlier verdict and declared "the interviews of the children were highly improper and utilized coercive and unduly suggestive methods."[71]

The phenomenon of recovered memories of traumatic childhood abuse raised a number of issues: how could such major traumatic events such as sexual abuse be forgotten? If traumas were forgotten, how can memories of them be recovered? Can people develop recollections of traumatic events that never occurred?[72] Most importantly, Did recovered memories reproduce actual events or were they products of therapists' suggestions? Psychologists, in particular, turned their attention toward empirical studies that attempted to answer these questions.

THE DOWNFALL OF THE RECOVERED MEMORY MOVEMENT

Proponents of recovered memory believed that the surge of traumatic cases that emerged in the 1980s and continued into the following decade reflected the growing recognition of genuine abuse that had been present, but had gone unreported, in previous eras. Many advocates regarded even the most preposterous tales of satanic ritual abuse as true because, according to Bass and Davis, "None of us want to believe such stories but for the sake of the survivors we must."[73]

As seemingly fantastic claims of abuse spread more widely and became a prominent topic of media attention, an opposition group emerged, which proposed that recovered traumatic memories were not so much uncovered as they were created by a combination of unstable patients, partisan clinicians, and credulous media portrayals. They echoed a long-standing history, dating to the nineteenth century, which indicated that suggestion, not trauma, was often the driving force behind the recognition of repressed memories. A student of Charcot's, Joseph Babinski, had demonstrated that hysterical symptoms often arose through patients' desires to please their therapists. In 1884, French physician Hippolyte Bernheim provided perhaps the first demonstration that clinicians could implant false traumatic memories. Bernheim told a hypnotized woman that she had witnessed a murder, which the woman subsequently reported to the police.[74] Likewise, in 1906 American physician James Jackson Putnam observed that Freud's techniques established a "dependence of the patient upon the physician which it may, in the end, be difficult to get rid of."[75] Sybil's florid presentations of her multiple personalities were the most obvious example of symptoms resulting from the suggestions of her therapist, Cornelia Wilbur. Noted psychiatrist Herbert Spiegel, who collaborated with Wilbur in Sybil's treatment, later called her case "an embarrassing phase of American psychiatry."[76]

Some instances of recovered memories involved patients who entered therapy without any knowledge of their early traumas but whose recollections emerged only during their clinical encounters.[77] Their therapists urged such patients to read or watch popular books and movies about childhood sexual abuse; they regarded signs of subsequent discomfort as indicators of earlier exploitation. They also had patients visualize scenes of molestation by family members. One patient, who later successfully sued her psychiatrist, "soon recovered memories of being molested by as many as fifty relatives, including both parents, both sets of grandparents, aunts, uncles, and great-grandparents."[78]

As the RMM became widely known through media reports, many women heard stories of recovered memories of abuse on television, read about them in magazines and books, and discussed them with their friends. They then sought sympathetic therapists who assured them that their symptoms likely indicated abuse. These clinicians colluded with patients in shared beliefs that the memories uncovered in therapy mirrored real childhood traumas. In these self-initiated cases, the process of recovering repressed memories was a mutual production between willing patients and their advocacy-oriented therapists. The resulting memories were less products of therapeutic suggestion than of clinicians reinforcing the expectations of their self-selected clients.

By the early 1990s a counterattack to the recovered memory movement had emerged from psychologists who were experts in the study of memory and were often allied with parents whose children had accused them of sexual abuse after uncovering repressed memories in therapy. These psychologists insisted that the premises of the recovered memory movement ran counter to virtually all scientific findings about how memory works. This evidence dated to the early twentieth century, when Harvard psychologist Hugo Münsterberg indicated that people could not know when their memories deceived them because both true and false recollections of past events had the same truthful qualities for those who experienced them.[79] From the point of view of these psychologists, the media, sympathetic interpersonal networks, and clinical advocates more than any actual childhood experiences created the traumatic memories uncovered in therapy. "The disorder may constitute a specific idiom of distress for some deeply troubled people who have been suitably prepared by the cultural environment," psychologist Daniel Schacter noted.[80]

A number of psychologists challenged each of the basic tenets of the recovered memory movement—that the most traumatic events are the ones most likely to be repressed, that the brain preserves traumatic memories with camera-like accuracy, and that repressed memories of abuse are always true. Their research contributed to the downfall of the RMM.

Severity and Repression

One of the recovered memory movement's core assumptions was that the most severe and continuous cases of abuse were *more* likely to be repressed than mundane and isolated incidents. This tenet stemmed from Janet's observations that hysterical patients could not integrate extremely intense shocks into their normal consciousness. For example, influential psychiatrist Lenore Terr contended that, while single episodes of abuse are typically remembered vividly, repeated abuse is commonly repressed.[81] Psychiatrist Colin Ross, another leading figure in the movement, characterized a typical case of repressed memory: "The sexual abuse usually starts before age five, lasts more than ten years, involves more than one perpetrator, and includes at least vaginal intercourse and fellatio."[82]

In contrast to this assumption, research consistently showed that the natural fading of the intensity of memories over time, rather than their active repression, accounts for the inability of people to recall traumas that occurred in the distant past. More severe traumas, however, were associated with stronger, not weaker, recall. Psychologists also found that repetition leads to improved, not loss of, memory for information.[83] Their studies found a strong positive correlation between the severity and repeated nature of the initial trauma and the vividness and endurance of memories of that trauma.

Although the RMM often invoked the experiences of Holocaust victims, this group intensely remembered their horrific traumas.[84] Even after the passage of many years, they showed a "remarkable degree of remembering" of their period of captivity.[85] Individuals who were victims of serious accidents, rapes, assaults, and other crimes, too, typically held detailed and accurate memories a number of years after their traumas had occurred. Traumatized people, far from having memory deficits, remembered their abuse all too well. Instead, they have an impaired ability to *forget* disturbing material.[86]

The Accuracy of Recovered Memories

Another principle of the recovered memory movement is that traumatic memories are literal recordings of reality that are embedded in brains at the time they occur. The shocks that generate them, however, are so severe that they cannot be assimilated into consciousness. Instead, they remain in the unconscious or subconscious in a pure, if inaccessible, state.[87]

Psychologists debunked the assertions that dissociated memories of traumatic events were accurately preserved in the brain. They found no evidence that people forget years of violent abuse that occurs after the age of two or so (infants younger than this age do not have the capacity to remember traumas). Most people can't remember experiences that occurred before age four or five.[88] Instead, their research supported Richard McNally's conclusion: "The notion that the mind protects itself by repressing or dissociating memories of trauma, rendering them inaccessible to awareness, is a piece of psychiatric folklore devoid of convincing empirical support."[89]

The contention that forgotten memories of childhood traumas remain in the same, pristine state as when they were originally experienced violates a number of principles about how memory operates. One is that the more time that has elapsed between some traumatic event and attempts to remember it, the less accurate the recollection is likely to be. Memories normally fade away, so people are increasingly unable to recall events with the passage of time. Natural processes of forgetting, not those of repression, account for why memories deteriorate over time. For example, almost everyone remembers traffic accidents after three months but over a quarter of victims fail to report experiencing the accident after nine to twelve months.[90]

Research also supported the principle that memories are not permanent and unalterable but require interpretation. Psychologist Daniel Schacter summarized: "We do not store judgment-free snapshots of our past experiences but rather hold on to the meaning, sense, and emotions these experiences provided us."[91] The mind is not like a video recorder that reproduces exactly what happened in the past. Instead, memories consist of how people recall early experiences in light of the interpretations they make in their current situations: "A neural network combines information in the present environment with patterns that have been stored in the past, and the resulting mixture of the two is what the network remembers," Schacter explained.[92]

Psychologists showed that the role of the highly emotionally charged therapeutic situation in which memory retrieval occurs is as important as or more important than the past events to which memories refer. One study compared three groups of individuals: those who had always remembered their abuse; those who recovered memories of abuse outside of therapy; and those who recovered memories of abuse during therapy.[93] While other people could corroborate 45 percent and 37 percent of memories in the first and second groups, not a single case of memories uncovered by suggestive therapeutic techniques was independently substantiated. "The analyst," Schacter stressed, "is a critical component of the retrieval setting who helps determine—not merely uncover—the form and content of the patient's memories."[94]

The recovered memory movement also ignored one of Freud's most insightful observations: many instances of childhood sexual abuse were *not* traumatic at the time they were experienced but only became so in light of later reinterpretations. Freud noted how many victims actually enjoyed sexual stimulation as young children, but only as teenagers became aware that these feelings stemmed from reprehensible situations.[95] Thus, later understandings have a tremendous impact on what eventually gets defined as traumatic. The "traumatic" aspects of many events that come to be defined as "abuse" are not intrinsic qualities of the events but construals stemming from interpretations that occur many years later.

Finally, in line with nineteenth-century critics, psychologists discredited hypnosis as a method for recovering accurate memories. Hypnosis often heightens patients' confidence that their memories are real, but no evidence shows that hypnosis-elicited memories are more accurate than memories that occur naturally. For example, thousands of patients remembered satanic ritual abuse while under hypnotic trances but not a single documented case of remembered satanic ritual abuse has been found to relate to real events.[96] "The discrepancy between evidential support and popularity could not be more striking," McNally concluded.[97]

Memory researchers thus showed how emotional and interpersonal forces in the present, including therapeutic suggestion, strongly shaped people's views of the past. Memory is far more subjective, interpretative, and constantly shifting than it is permanent, fixed, and objective.[98]

Belief in False Memories

Researchers also refuted another core principle of the RMM: patient recollections are almost always true. Instead, they indicated that memories are just as likely to involve distortions or outright falsehoods as they are to accurately reflect past occurrences. The best-known work stemmed from psychologist Elizabeth Loftus's research, which showed how memories do not precisely mirror past events but are easily subject to manipulation.[99] Loftus conducted a now-famous experiment with a fourteen-year-old boy, who read descriptions of four events that had happened in his childhood. One of these concerned a completely fabricated incident recounting how the boy had been lost in a shopping mall when he was five years old. Even after being informed that the occurrence had never happened, the boy continued to insist his memory still felt real to him. Many other studies have similarly found that people recall childhood experiences that are demonstrably false, such as spilling a punch bowl at a wedding, being hospitalized overnight, almost drowning, or being attacked by a vicious animal.[100] Overall, about a third of subjects believed that such implanted false memories of experiences that had never occurred were true.

Ironically, the recovered memory movement was responsible for stimulating much of the research that has greatly enhanced knowledge about how memory works. In thoroughgoing contrast to the tenets of this movement, a large body of evidence shows that memory is highly malleable in response to suggestions, that people can recover memories of events that never occurred, that memories naturally decay over time, that memories of past emotional traumas are inherently incomplete, constructed, and dependent on present states, and that hypnosis can produce compelling but utterly false memories. Other memories simply no longer exist to be recovered.[101]

The evidence regarding how memory works had no impact on recovered memory supporters. Herman, for example, dismissed these findings. Arguments against recovered memory, she wrote in 1997, are "ludicrously implausible." She continued: "Some attacks have been downright silly; many have been quite ugly. . . . They remind us also that moral neutrality in the conflict between victim and perpetrator is not an option."[102] Bass and Davis, too, were unconcerned with scientific findings. "Look," Bass claimed, "if we waited for scientific knowledge to catch up, we could just forget the whole thing. My ideas are not based on any scientific theories."[103] Terr, as well, claimed that experimental evidence about how memory works does not refute the claims of the RMM because "trauma sets up new rules for memory."[104] For such believers, recovered memories involved moral claims that empirical evidence could not refute.

Litigation against Recovered Memory Advocates

The decline of the recovered memory (and multiple personality) movement resulted more from litigation than from the findings of research psychologists. While recovered memory advocates disregarded or derided research about how memory works, they could not do the same with the growing number of lawsuits that were pursued against them. Most importantly, parents who were targets of their children's accusations of sexual abuse founded the False Memory Syndrome Foundation in 1992.[105] The FMSF mobilized a board composed of many professional experts in memory research. The confrontation between the debunkers and the believers in false memory syndrome was explicitly political and mostly played out in judicial proceedings.

The FMSF brought many lawsuits against recovered memory therapists. Sociologist Richard Ofshe and journalist Ethan Watters report that between 1993 and 1994 malpractice lawsuits against mental health professionals that involved recovered memories increased eight-fold, from 2 to 16 percent.[106] Courts increasingly came to question the reliability of recovered memories of early traumas. In one highly publicized case, psychiatrist Bennett Braun, a member of the *DSM-III-R* Task Force, settled one of his patient's lawsuits against him for nearly $11 million. This patient claimed that she was a priestess in a satanic cult that had, among other things, cannibalized 2,000 children a year and watched as she was raped by gorillas, panthers, and tigers at a zoo.[107] The judicial system, not professional organizations, became the enforcer of ethical practices.

The media took heed of legal developments and began to question the credibility of the RMM. The success of lawsuits against recovered memory therapists also led clinicians to rethink the techniques they used to encourage their patients to discover their hidden memories. Once therapists backed off of their promotion of recovered memories and the media questioned their reliability, people no longer newly recalled previously buried traumatic events. Insurance companies also stopped reimbursing long-term treatments for the condition. In a remarkably short time, the epidemic of recovered memories and associated traumatic disorders among women virtually disappeared. By the mid-1990s, the RMM had disintegrated.

The MPD diagnosis itself was abolished and renamed "dissociative identity disorder" (DID) in 1994 because, as the head of the relevant *DSM-IV* Work Group stated: "We wanted this condition to be regarded like any other mental disorder, and not like some weird, far-out, cultlike thing."[108] The text also noted how the condition could be the result of memories that "were subject to distortion" and that it occurred among individuals who were "especially vulnerable to suggestive influences."[109] DID failed to catch on, however, and therapists increasingly came to rely on PTSD as their diagnosis of choice for traumatic problems.[110] As psychiatrist Paul McHugh, one of the major critics of the recovered memory movement, presciently predicted at the time: "In but a few years we will all look back and be dumbfounded by the gullibility of the public in the late twentieth century and by the power of psychiatric assertions to dissolve common sense."[111]

CONCLUSION

The rapid rise of the recovered memory movement, as well as the associated multiple personality disorder movement, during the 1980s indicated the powerful role of suggestion in creating trauma-related diagnoses. More than any other mental illness, early memories of childhood traumas were products of therapeutic attention combined with the media's celebration and reinforcement of this telegenic condition. Once the iatrogenic nature of recovered memories became apparent, often within legal proceedings, they virtually disappeared from the mental health landscape.

Correspondingly, the rapid disappearance of patients who recovered memories of early abuse in the 1990s strongly implies that the epidemic of repressed childhood traumas during the preceding decade was a product of suggestion and not of real events. By the mid-1990s the recovered memory movement was in sharp decline, and by end of the decade "repressed memory syndrome was in disgrace."[112] From the vantage point of thirty years later, it seems that recovered memories were a product of cultural memes, social movements, and therapeutic suggestions.

The RMM directed patients to explore their distant pasts as a way of explaining their current problems. Instead of addressing recent stressors and difficulties, sufferers tagged long forgotten traumas perpetrated by their fathers or other relatives as being responsible for their existing mental disturbances. Once clinicians associated with the RMM discarded recovered memories as markers of traumas, they could use the far more acceptable PTSD diagnosis for their traumatized patients. Since the 1990s, post-traumatic stress disorder has become the unquestioned trope for characterizing the impact of traumas for women and men alike.

CHAPTER SIX

PTSD Becomes Ubiquitous

Twenty years ago posttraumatic stress was largely the preserve
of psychiatry. Today the language of trauma permeates everyday
discourse, television and radio talk, print journalism,
popular fiction, etc. The language of posttraumatic stress
is the Esperanto of global suffering.

Allan Young, *Journal of Nervous and Mental Disease*

"There are no unwounded soldiers in war"
(sign at Fort Hood coffeehouse)

Jerry Lembcke, *PTSD*

In 1966, the sociologist Philip Rieff published a book entitled *The
Triumph of the Therapeutic*.[1] It explored how the rise of therapeutic viewpoints had displaced religion as a key source of meaning in
Western societies. Therapy-oriented cultures venerate the feelings
of individuals above all other values. In contrast to past eras, when
faith-based beliefs bound sufferers to shared symbolic religious
systems, psychoanalysis and other therapeutic methods promoted
self-awareness as the preeminent ideal. Yet Rieff viewed members
of therapeutic cultures as fragile and vulnerable, with limited ca-

pacities to overcome their difficulties by themselves. They required the help of professional therapists, who supplanted spiritual authorities as the means for personal salvation. Rieff could not have known that the phenomenon he described was only in its infancy at the time. The culture he described now permeates the ways that people make sense of their disturbing feelings.

Therapeutic culture is a set of values that is promoted by organized interests—professional organizations, lay advocacy groups, and government officials. Large segments of the population have increasingly embraced its tenets. In particular, a marked growth in the number of mental health clinicians and the patients who use their services has occurred in recent decades. One major national survey, which showed that less than 1 percent of respondents sought professional help for mental health problems in 1957, reported that nearly 20 percent sought these services in 1996.[2] Around the time Rieff wrote, mental health organizations recorded about 1.2 million outpatient visits. This number increased to 2.8 million in 1979 and to 3.5 million in 1994.[3] By 2010, some 700,000 clinically trained mental health providers of all sorts were practicing in the United States.[4] They rarely impose labels of mental illness on resistant patients; instead, therapists and their clients participate in a shared culture of therapeutic values.

Although therapeutic cultures have existed in various forms since the late nineteenth century, a key difference between earlier eras and the present is that opposing institutions and beliefs no longer challenge them. In contrast to past eras, no health professional, regardless of his or her theoretical allegiance, considers mental illness to be a blameworthy condition. The media, as well, consistently presents positive portrayals of therapeutic values. Likewise, politicians on all sides generally unite in advocating compassionate attitudes toward the mentally ill. Most organized religious groups also embrace therapeutic viewpoints. Perhaps most importantly, in the past, norms of masculinity that resisted the open display of feelings and expressions of vulnerability checked the ability of therapeutic mentalities to gain broader societal dominance. Now, the culture of therapy celebrates men, not just women, who acknowledge their traumatic feelings and seek professional help for them. Therapeutic values currently permeate formerly male bastions, including professional athletics, the police, and emergency responders. Even the military, traditionally a citadel of antitherapeutic views, no longer stigmatizes psychically disturbed soldiers but has become a key participant in the therapeutic state.

TRAUMA CULTURE

Traumas are central to therapeutic narratives. Since Rieff wrote, the range of experiences that is considered to be traumatic and that can benefit from professional clinical assistance has expanded tremendously. From their delimited origins in combat, rape, horrific accidents, natural disasters, and other life-threatening situations, they have come to encompass such events as watching tragedies unfold on television, hearing news that a friend or relative has died, receiving unwelcome sexual attention, and at the extreme, reading novels with traumatic episodes. Studies have identified PTSD in people who have had wisdom teeth removed, given birth in uncomplicated deliveries, heard sexual jokes at work, discovered their spouse to be having an extramarital affair, or even watched a bad movie or TV program.[5] David Morris, one of the most insightful scholars of PTSD, notes: "As any trauma researcher will tell you, PTSD is everywhere today."[6]

The culture of trauma pervades social institutions. "Twenty years ago," anthropologist Allan Young observed in 2007, "posttraumatic stress was largely the preserve of psychiatry. Today, the language of trauma permeates everyday discourse, television and radio talk, print journalism, popular fiction, etc. The language of posttraumatic stress is the Esperanto of global suffering."[7] Schools and colleges provide one example. In 2016 the use of trigger warnings in classrooms became a major issue. These statements alert students who might be susceptible to PTSD to the potentially trauma-inducing nature of written material. One Rutgers student requested that an assignment requiring *The Great Gatsby* come with a warning stating, "suicide, domestic abuse and graphic violence."[8]

Trigger warnings testify to the great expansion of PTSD: reminders of racism, domestic violence, or sexual abuse can "trigger" memories of all sorts that make people vulnerable to painful flashbacks of traumatic experiences. In a widely quoted 2004 book, *Understanding Words That Wound*, cultural theorists Richard Delgado and Jean Stefancic's claims of the psychic impacts of hate speech echo those of wartime psychiatrists: "The immediate short-term harms of hate speech include rapid breathing, headaches, raised blood pressure, dizziness, rapid pulse rate, drug-taking, risk-taking behavior and even suicide."[9] During the 2016 presidential election, a group of Emory University students claimed to be "traumatized" when they found "Trump 2016" chalked on their campus sidewalks.[10] Trump's comments about women led to assertions such as, "Women told me they had flashbacks to hideous episodes in their past after the second presidential debate on 9 October, or couldn't sleep, or had nightmares."[11]

A cadre of supportive institutions bolsters the growing culture of trauma. Since the PTSD diagnosis emerged in the *DSM-III*, a largely autonomous profession that studies and treats trauma has arisen with its own ideology, journals, conferences, and training capacity. Their efforts became institutionalized with the establishment of the International Society for Traumatic Stress Studies in 1985 and its associated *Journal of Traumatic Stress* in 1988. Articles about PTSD in the medical literature doubled between 1985 and 1995 and then doubled again between 1995 and 2005. By 1999 more than 16,000 overall publications concerned PTSD.[12] The use of the term "PTSD" in books slowly grew during the 1980s, and then exploded by about 350 percent through 2008.[13] Trauma counselors became firmly embedded in schools, hospitals, corporations, the military, the judicial system, and disaster relief organizations. The Veterans Administration, which distributes billions of dollars for PTSD research, treatment, and benefits, is currently the second-largest department in the federal government.[14]

By the twenty-first century, the 150-year contention between those who associated PTSD with malingering or flawed character and those who saw it as the consequence of overpowering traumatic events was over: the medicalization of PTSD was complete. Regardless of whether the condition resulted from exposure to traumas or from vulnerability among those who were exposed, PTSD victims were not cowards, shirkers, or fortune hunters; they suffered from an illness that deserved compassion, treatment, and often, financial compensation. The *DSM* definition of PTSD is at the heart of trauma culture.

PTSD IN THE *DSM*

Changes in the criteria for post-traumatic stress disorder that are found in the diagnostic and statistical manuals since the *DSM-III* (1980) both reflected and stimulated the culture of trauma. As the previous chapter noted, the *DSM-III-R* (1986) substantially broadened the symptom criteria to incorporate forgotten, as well as intrusive, memories. The *DSM-IV* (1994), however, brought about the major expansion of the PTSD diagnosis. The initial *DSM-III* criteria had focused on extreme traumas that were "outside the range of normal human experience"; to qualify, such traumas had to "cause distress in almost everyone." The revised standard in the *DSM-IV* included all cases that the earlier definition had captured but added many other experiences, stipulating that "the person experienced, witnessed, or was confronted with events that involved actual or threatened death or serious injury, or a threat to the physical integrity of self or others," and that "the person's response involved intense fear, helplessness, or horror."[15]

These changes immensely broadened the boundaries of traumatic events to include not only those directly exposed to some trauma but also witnesses and even those "confronted with" information, such as a trauma unfolding on mass media. The "confronted with" criterion, in particular, extended the notion of exposure so widely that persons who were not even present at a traumatic event could potentially meet the diagnostic criteria. For example, someone who learns of the sudden and unexpected death of a close relative or that a friend has died from natural causes would meet the new stressor criterion. Even people who watched on television as a disaster occurred thousands of miles away could potentially be diagnosed with PTSD.[16]

The *DSM-IV* changed the nature of traumatic exposure in a second way. The requirement that the person's response involve "fear, helplessness, or horror" shifted the definitional criteria from the nature of the stressor to include the experience of the victim. Individual temperament, personality, and reactivity now entered into what defined an event as "traumatic" in the first place. This addition introduced a subjective element into the nature of the stressor itself, because only people who have a certain emotional reaction to the stressor are considered to have experienced a traumatic event. The *DSM-IV* thus expanded definitions of trauma both to include a great heterogeneity of events and to locate the nature of trauma within the individual as well as in the environment.[17]

The most recent revision of the manual, the *DSM-5* (2013), for the most part kept the PTSD diagnostic criteria intact. It tightened the most expansive aspect of the previous criteria by removing the most subjective aspect of the *DSM-IV* diagnosis: intense emotional reactions were no longer a definitional component of PTSD. It also specified that witnessing some catastrophe through the media does not qualify as a traumatic event, so that traumas must involve "exposure to actual or threatened death, serious injury, or sexual violence."[18] However, the *DSM-5* expanded the criteria by adding a category of exposure for people such as police or social workers who had repeated exposure to reports of traumatic experiences and by lowering the diagnostic threshold for children and adolescents.

The various editions of the *DSM* manuals, especially the *DSM-III-R* and *DSM-IV*, broadened the PTSD diagnosis from its delineated origin in the conditions of combat veterans and a small number of other traumatized groups to encompass virtually the entire population. Their diluted stressor criterion helped create a vast array of pathology that extended far beyond previous conceptions of PTSD. They also paved the way for a reconciliation of viewpoints that in the past had stressed either exposure or vulnerability as reasons for developing PTSD.

Reconciling Exposure and Vulnerability

The rise of therapeutic culture, combined with the *DSM* revisions to the PTSD diagnosis, thoroughly reoriented the controversy over whether traumas emerged because of exposure to traumatic events or because of predisposing vulnerabilities to them. Throughout the history of PTSD, this issue had dominated debates about the causes of PTSD. In previous eras, defendants in court cases involving railway spine sought to avoid liability by assigning fault to the weakness or malingering of plaintiffs, who attributed their psychic symptoms to the shock of accidents themselves; many military physicians faulted weak-willed men for succumbing to shell shock or combat neuroses, whereas others emphasized the stress of battle itself; governments tried to deflect compensatory obligations for combat-related breakdowns onto preexisting conditions, unlike pension seekers, who asserted that wartime conditions explained their symptoms.

The veterans and their psychiatric allies who established the purely exposure-oriented focus of PTSD in the *DSM-III* were responding to this long-standing association of personal vulnerability with blame for psychic impairments. The rise of trauma culture, however, rendered superfluous the issue of the relative weight of exposure and vulnerability as explanations of PTSD. Anyone who displayed signs of PTSD, regardless of the reason, was entitled to claim the status of a traumatized victim.

During the period between the 1940s and 1970s, the sociocultural focus of the mental health professions had led the brain to mostly disappear as a focus of study for traumatic conditions. The *DSM-III*'s purely environmental turn left no room for debates, which had dominated discussions of the causes of railway spine and shell shock, between those who assumed that powerful external stressors could create neurological changes among all people who were exposed to them, and those who emphasized that traumatic psychic disturbances were only likely to emerge among victims who were already predisposed to develop mental illnesses. Its criteria for PTSD had a distinct and unambiguous etiology, originating in an external stressor that was likely to have serious psychic impacts among all people who were exposed to it, not just the biologically susceptible.

The emergence of neuroscience as a dominant force in psychiatry and psychology in the 1970s changed the terms of the dispute between advocates of exposure and those of vulnerability as the major reason behind the development of stressor-related conditions. By 1980, the stressor-based nature of the *DSM-III*'s PTSD diagnosis was in considerable tension with the basic assumptions of the psychiatric profession, which had come to refocus on brain-based aspects of mental disturbances. Out of the hundreds of diagnoses found in the *DSM-III*, PTSD almost uniquely emphasized environmental causation. This stressor-based condition did not mesh well with the new biological model that was already beginning to dominate the profession when the *DSM-III* was published and that was clearly ascendant in it by the early 1990s.[19]

Psychiatrists and neuropsychologists were rapidly turning toward examining the brain as the locus of disorders, emphasizing individual susceptibilities and predispositions. "Overall," psychologist Marilyn Bowman and neuroscientist Rachel Yehuda summarized, "research demonstrates that PTSD is best understood as the periodic expression of long-standing dispositions that often are risk factors for both threatening exposures and subsequent dysfunctions."[20] The contribution that brain-based approaches would make toward understanding PTSD would be diminished if events triggered symptoms in previously unimpaired individuals. Reconciliation between the stressor-based conception of PTSD and the brain-based focus of psychiatry became inevitable as neuroscience increasingly became the major source of validation for legitimate mental disturbances.

The *DSM-IV* criteria provided the means for integrating the focus on exposure to traumatic events with the study of individual proneness to them. As noted, they incorporated subjective definitions of and responses to traumas into the definition of what a "trauma" was. This insured that factors having to do with individual responses to events as well as the events themselves would have explanatory importance. "The more we broaden the category of traumatic stressors," psychologist Richard McNally asserted, "the less credibly we can assign causal significance to a given stressor in itself and the more weight we must place on personal vulnerability factors."[21] Following nineteenth- and early twentieth-century models, studies began reemphasizing how personal predispositions helped account for the emergence of PTSD.

Trauma researchers have increasingly placed their faith in biological findings as a way of legitimating post-traumatic stress disorder as a "real" mental disorder.[22] Some neuroscientists claim that brain scanning techniques, including magnetoencephalography (MEG) or magnetic resonance imaging (MRI), can identify the neuroelectrical correlates of PTSD with 90 percent accuracy.[23] Thousands of studies now examine the relationship of such factors as levels of cortisol and adrenalin, the size of various brain regions, or patterns of brain activation in response to traumatic stimuli to the development of PTSD. The explosion of neuroscientific studies in psychiatry and psychology provides a physiological underpinning and thus potential validation for PTSD by showing how memories are literally part of the brain.[24] The neuroscientific turn has moved from the laboratory to social institutions: for example, the federal government now requires that all institutions of higher education train their staff about the effects of "neurobiological change" in victims of sexual assault, so that they can conduct "trauma-informed" investigations and judgments.[25] "The narrative of trauma has become less about politics and inner psychic conflict and more about stress hormones and the chemical dance of synapses," David Morris summarizes.[26]

By the beginning of the twenty-first century, the controversy over whether exposure or vulnerability leads to PTSD had largely evaporated. Traumatologists take for granted that traumatic events produce huge levels of pathology and that brain-based defects account for which particular individuals exposed to traumas will develop PTSD. In contrast to earlier historical periods, advocates of both externally and internally focused explanations champion the legitimacy of PTSD diagnoses. Both sides strive to identify and treat as many victims as possible among the exposed and the susceptible alike.

TRAUMAS IN THE GENERAL POPULATION

Definitional changes in the *DSM* criteria led to corresponding increases in the proportion of the population who suffered "traumas." A notable study using the *DSM-III-R* criteria among a large sample in Detroit in the late 1980s found that 39 percent of residents had been exposed to some traumatic event.[27] The most renowned community study of mental disorders, the National Co-Morbidity Survey (NCS), also used the *DSM-III-R* criteria in its survey of nearly 6,000 respondents across the United States during the early 1990s.[28] It found that over 60 percent of men and over 50 percent of women reported at least one traumatic event, the most common being witnessing someone else being badly injured or killed. Community research using the even more expansive *DSM-IV* criteria showed that traumas were virtually ubiquitous in the population. One study of more than 2,000 residents of southeast Michigan in the mid-1990s indicated that about 90 percent had been exposed to some traumatic event, nearly a 60 percent increase over studies using the prior *DSM-III-R* criteria. The most common trauma was the sudden, unexpected death of a close friend or relative, which accounted for one-third of all traumatic events. "Almost everyone," the authors concluded, "has experienced a PTSD-level event."[29] Trauma had moved from battlefield, disaster, or rape situations into the realm of everyday life.

Levels of PTSD itself also increased dramatically. The initial studies, which used the original *DSM-III* definition, found rates of about 1 percent or less in the general population. Subsequent research employing the expanded *DSM-III-R* criteria showed significantly elevated rates of PTSD. The NCS reported that about 8 percent of respondents suffered from PTSD at some point in their lives. The Detroit study indicated a similar rate, of about

9 percent.[30] Anthropologist Allan Young noted that in the later studies, the lifetime prevalence for women was nine times higher and for men thirty-five times higher than in the Epidemiologic Catchment Area study in 1980![31]

Community studies also indicated the gendered nature of trauma. Although men were somewhat more likely than women to experience traumas, women reported about twice as much PTSD as men.[32] Rape was especially traumatic—80 percent of female rape victims suffered from PTSD soon after the assault. Sexual violence against women was not just associated with much higher risks of PTSD but also with longer-lasting symptoms of PTSD.[33]

These studies also showed, however, that most cases that met criteria for PTSD dissipated in a relatively short time, usually without any therapeutic intervention. For example, about 66 percent of female victims of nonsexual assaults qualified for a PTSD diagnosis ten days after the assault. By one month only 45 percent qualified, and by one year only 12 percent met PTSD criteria. Even the PTSD symptoms of most rape victims, who generally fared worse than sufferers of any other type of traumatic event, gradually declined over time. Almost all women experienced PTSD in the immediate aftermath of the rape and nearly three-quarters suffered from this condition one month later. While half still had PTSD three months later, the condition remained in one-quarter of victims a year after a rape. Although sizable minorities of trauma victims develop chronic conditions, the typical course of PTSD is for gradually decreasing severity and natural recovery over time.[34]

Studies in the late 1980s and 1990s indicated the widespread presence of traumas and resulting PTSD in communities. They also showed the influence of changing definitions about what constitutes a "trauma" on the resulting rates of traumatic events and their psychic consequences. The major factor, however, propelling traumas into public consciousness was research about the psychological costs of collective disasters.

COLLECTIVE DISASTERS

Before the 1980s, little research had been done on the psychic impacts of shared traumas in civilian populations. The best-known studies were conducted during World War II among residents of London who faced German air attacks. In contrast to the expectations of psychiatrists, who predicted a massive outbreak of traumatic neuroses in the population, the incidence of such cases was "astonishingly small."[35] Prominent psychologist Irving Janis noted that "the reactions of most people generally subsided within one-quarter of an hour after the end of the bombing attack."[36] Indeed, admissions to psychiatric hospitals actually declined during this period. Researchers attributed the psychological resilience of civilians to the sense of common purpose to endure attacks and to defeat the Nazis that prevailed at the time. "Most important of all," historian Ben Shephard reports, "civilians were able to keep around them their family and home, their friends and community, the bastions of their emotional security."[37]

American sociologists who engaged in disaster research between the end of World War II and the 1980s also focused on how shared calamities often increased social cohesion.[38] Disaster researchers viewed catastrophes that affected mass populations as structural problems requiring community mobilization and solidarity, rather than as threats to individual psyches. They emphasized the resilience, not the psychic susceptibilities, of people who faced adversities such as floods, earthquakes, and hurricanes. The behavior of people in the aftermath of disaster contradicted the belief that disasters led to widespread trauma, weakness, and vulnerability. Rebecca Solnit summarizes the findings of disaster research at the time: "The prevalent human nature in disaster is resilient, resourceful, generous, emphatic, and brave."[39]

Disaster research underwent a major reorientation after 1980 as the growing influence of trauma culture subsumed collective disasters into the realm of mental health problems. Widely publicized studies of human and natural disasters trumpeted the psychic damage, including post-traumatic stress disorder, which these traumas wrought. One review uncovered 284 studies of PTSD after disasters that were published between 1980 and 2007.[40] This research indicated that about 17 percent of people were exposed to disasters at some point in their life. It showed widely varying rates of resultant PTSD, ranging from 3.7 percent to 60 percent in the first two years after the event.[41] For example, 34 percent of adults injured in the 1994 Oklahoma City terrorist bombing reported PTSD six months later.[42] However, these studies also showed that PTSD symptoms rapidly declined after disasters in about 80 percent of samples.[43] Another consistent finding was that victims with prior mental health problems were especially likely to show chronic postdisaster disorders.[44]

Before the turn of the century knowledge of the extensive literature on the psychic effects of disasters was usually limited to the research community. The terrorist attacks on September 11, 2001, drove the psychological consequences of disasters into public consciousness. This event became by far the most studied collective trauma to date. Contemporaneous and nonstop news coverage of the carnage meant that the whole population of the nation (indeed, of much of the world)—not just those who were directly exposed to the attack—was "confronted with" a potentially traumatic event and so met the *DSM-IV* criteria for a stressor that could lead to PTSD.

The assumptions and expectations of trauma culture permeated the initial reaction to the attacks. Immediately after the destruction of the Twin Towers, thousands of mental health professionals rushed to the scene.[45] A reporter estimated that the 9,000 mental health counselors who arrived outnumbered the quantity of victims by a factor of three.[46] One psychiatrist's expectation was representative: "[There will be] huge increases in the prevalence of traumatic grief, depression, posttraumatic stress disorder and substance abuse in the New York City metropolitan at the least. This is an unprecedented disaster, and its psychiatric toll will be enormous."[47] James Nininger, then president of the New York State Psychiatric Association, wrote in the *New York Times* shortly after the disaster: "The true scope of the psychiatric problems will be seen not just over the ensuing months, but over years, and not only among those who were at ground zero or who lost, or feared that they had lost, a family member or friend but also among those who viewed the horrific scenes on TV."[48] The concern for mental health was strong enough that emergency personnel in New York City were required to participate in mental health treatment.[49] The Federal Emergency Management Agency (FEMA) spent $132 million on mental health services following September 11.[50]

Initially, it did appear that the terrorist attacks had led to widespread psychic damage. An early study taken a few days after them asked 560 respondents from across the country whether they experienced five symptoms of PTSD: "Feeling very upset when something reminds you of what happened? Repeated, disturbing memories, thoughts, or dreams about what happened? Having difficulty concentrating? Trouble falling or staying asleep? Feeling irritable or having angry outbursts?" Forty-four percent of those surveyed reported at least one "substantial" symptom, and virtually everyone (90 percent) experienced at least "a little bit" of a symptom. Over half of respondents said that at least one of their children was upset by the attacks. This study concluded that over 40 percent of Americans had symptoms of stress that "are unlikely to disappear soon."[51]

In fact, despite dire predictions that 9/11 would result in an enormous amount of lasting PTSD, rates dropped precipitously soon after the attacks. Studies showed that the 7.5 percent of Manhattan residents who suffered from PTSD one month after the event sharply declined to just 1.7 percent and 0.6 percent at four and six months, respectively, after the attacks.[52] This meant that more than 90 percent of persons who originally qualified for PTSD diagnoses no longer met the criteria for this condition after six months.[53] In the country at large, overall distress levels were within normal range one to two months after the attacks.[54] The almost immediate "recovery" of most people who were not directly affected by the attacks calls into question whether they ever had a traumatic disorder in the first place. In addition, rates of psychiatric disturbances, suicide, and violent crime dropped immediately after 9/11 and remained low six months later.[55]

The rapid decline in symptoms cannot be attributed to successful treatment efforts: despite predictions to the contrary, no rise in treatment rates occurred after 9/11. "Most people recover from acute symptoms within 3 months posttrauma, even if they do not receive any treatment," psychologists Richard McNally, Richard Bryant, and Anke Ehlers summarized.[56] Indeed, 7.6 percent of people used mental health services in the month after the attack compared to 8.6 percent in the month before the attack.[57] Nearly 90 percent of persons who sought mental health services after 9/11 had already been in treatment before the attacks. Most of the millions of dollars allocated for mental health services remained unspent because few people sought such therapy. Initial diagnoses of PTSD, spurred by the assumptions of trauma culture, seem to have reflected natural, transitory responses to a highly disturbing experience rather than a mental disorder. "New York City residents," psychiatrist Sally Satel concluded, "affirmed the general human response to crisis: reliance on traditional social institutions of community, family, and faith. Mental health professionals sorely underestimated their fortitude."[58]

Despite the evidence that 9/11 had few lasting psychic consequences, the assumptions of trauma culture continued to prevail in subsequent disasters. For example, after Hurricane Katrina hit the Gulf Coast in 2005, FEMA provided $52 million for crisis counseling.[59] Expectations of composure and resilience in the face of trauma had been transformed into victimhood and psychic vulnerability. "That disaster victims—or the victims of any trauma—require mental health assistance has become a commonplace in the early 21st century," historian Andrew Morris observed.[60]

In a survey of the early literature on community studies in 1987, epidemiologist Naomi Breslau and psychiatrist Glenn Davis concluded: "Literature on the effects of the Vietnam war and civilian disasters indicates that emotional disturbance (other than transient immediate reactions) is *not* a common consequence of these 'extreme' stressors."⁶¹ Rising rates of PTSD in community and disaster studies since that time do not stem from the presence of a more traumatized population or from the greater ability of researchers to identify traumatic disorders. Instead, they are the product of the expectations of a therapeutic culture that assumes disaster victims will succumb to traumatic stressors and will need mental health services.

THE MILITARY

The impact of therapeutic culture has been especially apparent within military institutions. As previous chapters indicated, for the past hundred years combat was linked with psychological trauma, whether through "shell-shock" in World War I, "combat neuroses" in World War II, or "PTSD" after Vietnam. Nevertheless, substantial numbers of military personnel refused to acknowledge the often dire psychic consequences of war. Officers commonly regarded military psychiatrists as either enablers of cowardly behavior or allies in the struggle to get impaired soldiers back into combat as soon as possible. As the conflict over the insertion of PTSD into the *DSM-III* illustrated, as late as the 1970s psychologically wounded veterans had to make extensive efforts against strong opposition to have their conditions recognized. In large part, the military's antagonism to traumatic psychic conditions resulted from its intrinsic emphasis on the traditionally masculine values of physical toughness, suppression of painful emotions, and insensitivity to discomfort (for male and female soldiers alike). By the twentieth-first century, however, the military had come to fully participate in therapeutic culture.

Rates of Psychological Casualties

Chapter 4 described how the initial studies among Vietnam veterans showed relatively low rates of PTSD. In the late 1980s Congress commissioned a study of PTSD among this group, the National Vietnam Veterans' Readjustment Study (NVVRS). This report found far higher amounts of PTSD than earlier research: at the time the study was conducted, about twenty years after the war's most intense fighting had ended, 15 percent of veterans met full diagnostic criteria for PTSD and an additional 11 percent had significant symptoms of the condition. The NVVRS also indicated that at some point after the war about 31 percent of men met full diagnostic criteria for PTSD and an additional 22.5 percent had partial PTSD.[62] These figures generated considerable suspicion because only about 15 percent of military forces in Vietnam had been in combat, with 15 percent more in supportive combat roles. If the study's findings were to be believed, then virtually every one of these personnel suffered from PTSD.

The rates of PTSD the NVVRS claimed to find were orders of magnitude beyond those found in previous studies. PTSD occurred seven times more often than in the earlier CDC Veterans Experience Study. The large number of PTSD cases that persisted so long after combat had ended also conflicted with studies of other contemporaneous wars. For example, less than 2 percent of Israeli veterans of the Yom Kippur War of 1973 still had a PTSD diagnosis thirty years later.[63] Another puzzle the NVVRS findings raised was that, in contrast to previous studies, rates of PTSD actually increased rather than declined over time.[64]

A number of skeptics claimed that the high rates of PTSD that arose so long after the war's end were more likely to indicate changes associated with the rise of trauma culture than with genuine increases in the number of cases of PTSD. One noted that "the Vietnam veteran is more a victim of his times, of the post–World War II culture and its values than of the Vietnam War itself."[65] Another commented that the results led him "to wonder how much we are dealing with the sequelae of post combat belief, expectation, explanation and attribution rather than the sequelae of combat itself."[66] For critics, the huge rates of PTSD the NVVRS reported indicated the extent to which the idea of the psychologically damaged Vietnam veteran had penetrated cultural expectations and influenced self-reported recollections of symptoms.

Doubt about the NVVRS findings led to an intensive reanalysis of a subsample of 260 of the original 1,200 men.[67] This subsequent study showed readjusted rates of PTSD that varied from 9 to 12 percent of veterans with current conditions and from 19 to 22.5 percent with lifetime conditions, numbers that were about 40 percent lower than the original estimates. Another reanalysis of the same data, which required that symptoms lead to at least moderate difficulties in functioning, found that prevalence had dropped by 65 percent from the original levels.[68]

Despite the controversy over the NVVRS, its findings of such high rates of PTSD were one reason the military changed its assumptions about how it should respond to the psychic results of combat.[69] Its mental health personnel expected that the Persian Gulf, Iraq, and Afghanistan Wars would result in high levels of PTSD. They embraced the view that PTSD is a widespread condition in wartime, that all soldiers can be potential victims, and that affected soldiers require treatment for it. Moreover, they assumed that PTSD would not be a time-limited condition but would often result in long-term consequences.[70] As a result, the military spent hundreds of millions of dollars for research about PTSD and traumatic brain disorders.[71] Mental health professionals gained a much stronger presence and higher prestige within the military; they are now widely esteemed and applauded for their service.[72]

Many studies examined levels of PTSD among veterans returning from the Persian Gulf, Iraq, and Afghanistan Wars.[73] The initial research about the impact of the 1991 Gulf War indicated that only about 3 percent of veterans reported PTSD immediately after the war. Two years later, however, this number had increased to about 8 percent.[74] These relatively low rates might reflect the limited amount of combat in and quick resolution of this conflict. Studies conducted during the 2000s, after the Iraq and Afghanistan Wars, reported far higher numbers—between 15 percent and 20 percent—of veterans with PTSD.[75] One major examination found that 25 percent of more than 100,000 veterans who returned from these wars received some mental health diagnosis; 13 percent were diagnosed with PTSD.[76] Another study of more than 100,000 veterans who were enrolled in the VA health system showed that over 20 percent had received PTSD diagnoses.[77]

PTSD was the single most common mental health condition, representing more than half of all mental health diagnoses. It was also linked to marital instability, problems with spouses, and domestic violence.[78] Curiously, about half of soldiers suffering from PTSD reported having this condition *before* they deployed to Iraq.[79]

Suicide, often linked to PTSD, also drew much attention from researchers and the media. Echoing the aftermath of the Vietnam War, front-page stories in newspapers around the country depicted suicidal (and homicidal) vets ravaged by PTSD.[80] Suicide rates among soldiers who served in Iraq and Afghanistan doubled between 2004 and 2009. Notably, however, suicides tripled among soldiers who were never deployed on the battlefield.[81] Another study reported that, "remarkably, nearly half of the soldiers with a history of lifetime suicide attempts reported that their first attempt occurred prior to enlistment."[82] Such findings indicated that preexisting vulnerabilities, as well as combat-related traumas, were behind many suicides and suicide attempts among veterans.

Responses to Psychological Casualties

Despite the far greater sensitivity to post-traumatic stress disorder within the armed services, the services' responses to affected soldiers are bifurcated. The military's traditional suspicion of invisible psychological injuries is still strong for soldiers on active duty. One soldier reported: "They told us in basic [training], 'Anything that's not life, limb, or eyesight, suck it up. If you say you're hurt, we're gonna assume you're faking.'"[83] Especially for personnel who plan to reenlist, PTSD diagnoses remain stigmatizing; they can raise questions about their bearers' suitability for future combat and stymie promotions.

The major change in the military's response to PTSD involves veterans who have returned home and are leaving or have already left active duty. All such soldiers, not just the predisposed, are thought to be in danger of developing PTSD. "There are no unwounded soldiers in war," a sign at a Fort Hood coffeehouse proclaims.[84] Indeed, unlike previous wars, in which the military used screening to detect mental health problems before soldiers entered service, the military now attempts to screen all *returning* veterans for postwar mental health problems and to refer those deemed at-risk to mental health interventions.[85] To this end, the VA has developed public awareness campaigns that actively pursue veterans who might have PTSD.[86] In addition, while in the past most traumatic conditions were expected to be short-lived, assumptions of chronicity are common. "There is a major health crisis facing those men and women who have served our nation in Iraq and Afghanistan," a major study concluded. "Unless they receive appropriate and effective care for these mental health conditions, there will be long-term consequences for them and for the nation."[87]

A wide variety of treatments for PTSD have emerged for returning soldiers. Drug therapies, which have been commonplace throughout the history of stress-related conditions, are still widely employed to manage combat stress and its aftermath. The pharmaceutical industry, however, has been unable to develop any drug that specifically targets PTSD. The SSRI (selective serotonin reuptake inhibitor) Zoloft is now the most widely used drug for PTSD, although there is little rhyme or reason to prescribing practices.[88] As one soldier noted, "As far as medications go, man, they throw so many of them at you and then hope to God one of them sticks."[89] The findings from a study of more than 186,000 veterans of the Iraq and Afghanistan Wars confirm this observation. Although none had diagnoses of schizophrenia or bipolar disorder, 35,000 received prescriptions for antipsychotic medication.[90]

Drugs are often used in combination with a variety of treatments, including exposure therapy, eye movement desensitization, and virtual reality, all of which are based on the principles of cognitive behavioral therapy. Prolonged exposure therapy, which regards avoidance as the central problem for PTSD sufferers, is the most prominent.[91] To allow for adequate processing of traumatic memories, it presents reminders of traumatic events in gradually increasing intensity until patients become habituated to the trauma. In 2008 an Institute of Medicine (IoM) panel concluded that exposure therapies are effective, and the VA has fully embraced them.[92]

Nevertheless, exposure therapy and other cognitive approaches have also drawn sharp criticism. Some researchers claim that PTSD symptoms worsen every time someone recalls a traumatic event because recollections trigger stress hormones that accompany painful memories, so emotions become more vivid with each subsequent recall.[93] Well-known PTSD researcher Bessel van der Kolk calls exposure therapy "among the worst possible treatments" for trauma.[94] Many sufferers don't like them. "Traditional medical approaches generally rely on drugs and controlled re-experiencing of trauma, called exposure therapy. But this combination has proved so unpopular that many veterans quit before finishing or avoid it altogether," a *New York Times* article concluded in 2016.[95] Consequently, exposure treatment has the highest dropout rate of any treatment.

Such conflicting assessments typify evaluations of treatments for PTSD. No drug or psychotherapeutic technique is reliably effective in treating this condition.[96] As one review concludes, "Conventional western psychiatric treatment along the lines used to treat other serious mental disorders—drugs, groups, therapy, in-patient facilities and so on—has not led to a record of undisputed therapeutic success for traumatized veterans."[97] Indeed, a study at the National Center for PTSD found that a four-month program of intensive inpatient care made patients' symptoms worse.[98] The 2008 IoM panel concluded: "At this time, we can make no judgment about the effectiveness of most psychotherapies or about any medications in helping patients with PTSD."[99] The disappointing results of mainstream psychological and drug therapies have led to the emergence of a potpourri of "treatments" for PTSD, including fishing, swimming with sharks, yoga, horseback riding, vision quests, and parrot husbandry, among many others.[100]

Questions remain about the extent to which aggressive efforts to identify and treat soldiers who are presumed to have PTSD actually identify disordered conditions and help the individuals so labeled. The intensity of the painful psychic impacts of traumatic events often naturally remits over time, especially when people have supportive resources that help them adjust to their experiences.[101] For example, an army report noted that the high rates of apparent mental disorder present in those returning from combat assignments decrease almost to baseline rates of those garrisoned at US military bases after about twenty-four months, and fully to baseline by thirty to thirty-six months, suggesting that most symptoms classified as PTSD remit on their own with time.[102] "Just as with a course of grief," psychiatrist Paul McHugh observes, "the most disturbing psychological symptoms gradually fade away, leaving the subject with some enduring sense of loss, the occasional bad dream, and perhaps some reluctance to revisit locations or arenas where the shock was experienced."[103]

The centrality of the PTSD diagnosis has led to intensely psychological approaches to treatment that differ in significant ways from past military responses. In particular, they neglect the bodily aspects of traumas that Abram Kardiner had called "physioneuroses." Trauma specialist Bessel van der Kolk emphasizes that PTSD is more of a bodily than a cognitive process: "Trauma has nothing whatsoever to do with cognition. It has to do with your body being reset to interpret the world as a dangerous place."[104] Prominent military psychiatrist Charles Hoge also notes how a central problem that returned veterans face involves the thoroughgoing need to undo the physiological responses to combat that veterans have previously gone through, which includes adjustment to prolonged extreme stress, chronic sleep restriction, and reversal of circadian cycles.[105]

Anthropologist Kenneth MacLeish's fieldwork at Fort Hood, Texas, supports these contentions. Soldiers identified unwanted, preconscious bodily sensitivity to signs of violence and danger as the major aspect of their current responses to past combat experiences.[106] While in Iraq or Afghanistan their bodies were in a constant state of activation, which persisted when they returned to the United States. MacLeish describes a typical case: "You're going about your business at Fort Hood, and you hear a helicopter or the sunny-day thunder of artillery fire rumbling in from the ranges, and before you even realize you heard it your guts turn to ice, your palms get clammy, and your whole body is arched and alert, ready to go." In contrast to the diagnostic emphasis on conscious memories of trauma, the soldiers that MacLeish studied reported "a direct line from sensory stimulus to neuromotor response, bypassing consciousness, thought, and interpretation."[107] Such responses resemble Kardiner's physioneuroses far more than the current mentalistic PTSD diagnosis, which emphasizes memory and cognition.

The focus on PTSD as the primary result of combat has also suppressed interest in the problems stemming from the social dislocations that veterans face. The need for social support, strong familial relationships, and employment opportunities were central to the rehabilitation literatures that emerged after World Wars I and II, when "a job and a girl" were seen as the optimal requirements for readjustment to civilian life.[108] From this perspective, the label "post-traumatic stress disorder" can divert attention from the sorts of things that returning veterans most need help with: negotiating complicated bureaucracies, finding employment and social services, reintegrating with families and friends, and coping with naturally distressing memories. In addition, PTSD labels can sometimes provide incentives for remaining disabled.

The Role of Compensation

The impact of providing compensation to people with traumatic diagnoses has been a controversial subject since the nineteenth century. Debates during the era of railway spine involved the issue of whether the rewards from traumatic diagnoses could themselves lead to chronicity. Before the Vietnam War, military psychiatrists believed that combat-related symptoms would rarely endure unless they were related to underlying predisposing conditions, or they resulted in rewards. Military physicians assumed that diagnoses could reinforce, stabilize, and perpetuate symptoms because if symptoms disappeared, so would compensation for them. Indeed, anthropologist Erin Finley predicts that "explosive consequences" would result if some treatment proved able to cure PTSD.[109]

By the twenty-first century, the general acceptance of therapeutic culture meant that no stigma accrued to veterans (and others) who received PTSD diagnoses. Yet, assessments are still entirely dependent on self-reported symptoms that are impossible to verify. By the 1990s, PTSD had become such a well-known condition that now virtually all veterans know what answers to give to achieve their desired goal (whether to receive or not to receive a PTSD label). Those who want to remain in the service and avoid getting diagnoses that enter their military records can easily deny having symptoms related to PTSD. Others, who are motivated to receive a diagnosis that can bring them disability pensions and other resources, are eager to report many symptoms.[110] The varying social consequences that the diagnosis entails help shape who will or will not have PTSD.

During the mid-1990s and through the following decades, rates of treated PTSD among veterans rose to unprecedented levels. Applications for PTSD-related compensation from veterans of the Iraq and Afghanistan Wars far exceeded those from earlier periods.[111] Between 2000 and 2013 the number of veterans in the VA system who received benefits for PTSD claims rose from about 134,000 to more than 650,000.[112] By the end of 2012, almost half of the 700,000 veterans of the Iraq and Afghanistan Wars had filed disability claims with the VA for all reasons, and 85 percent of these were receiving benefits. This compares to just 11, 16, and 21 percent, respectively, of veterans of World War II, Vietnam, and the Persian Gulf War.[113] These rates are much higher than those seen among personnel from other countries who fought in the same war. For example, only 3 percent of UK soldiers compared to 13 percent of US military personnel reported PTSD after the Iraq War.[114]

Interestingly, the increasing level of post-traumatic stress disorder claims since the mid-1990s was found not only among members of the armed forces who served in the Gulf, Iraq, and Afghanistan Wars but also among Vietnam veterans whose military service had ended thirty or more years earlier. Indeed, the rate of growth in use of VA mental health services for PTSD was five times greater for Vietnam-era veterans than for Gulf-era veterans.[115] In thorough contrast to previous wars and other disasters,

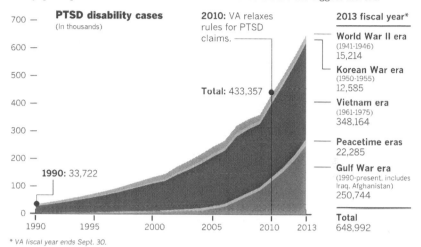

A steep rise in PTSD

The number of veterans on the disability rolls for post-traumatic stress disorder has nearly quintupled since 2000. Vietnam and the recent wars are the biggest drivers.

PTSD disability cases
(In thousands)

700 —
600 —
500 —
400 —
300 —
200 —
100 —
0 —

1990   1995   2000   2005   2010   2013

1990: 33,722

2010: VA relaxes rules for PTSD claims.

Total: 433,357

2013 fiscal year*

World War II era
(1941-1946)
15,214

Korean War era
(1950-1955)
12,585

Vietnam era
(1961-1975)
348,164

Peacetime eras
22,285

Gulf War era
(1990-present, includes Iraq, Afghanistan)
250,744

Total
648,992

* VA fiscal year ends Sept. 30.

Source: Department of Veterans Affairs. Graphics reporting by Alan Zarembo.
Thomas Suh Lauder / @latimesgraphics

in which rates of PTSD sharply declined with the passage of time, compensation-seeking among Vietnam War veterans exploded as the number of years since the war had ended accumulated. The numbers of such veterans who applied for disability related to PTSD expanded precipitously during the twenty-first century. Rates of Vietnam veterans receiving compensation for PTSD increased far more than those for veterans getting disability for all other health problems.[116]

Did the upsurge of PTSD diagnosis among veterans result from a genuine rise in the numbers of long-delayed conditions or from treatment-seekers who were deeply immersed in the culture of PTSD and who knew what responses were likely to obtain compensation? Unlike physical wounds, symptoms of PTSD are self-reported, invisible, and unverifiable. Mental health personnel historically believed that symptoms of PTSD are "subjective, easily coached, and easily simulated."[117] According to one recent report, in online forums, "veterans trade tips on how to behave in their disability evaluations. Common advice: Dress poorly and don't shower, refuse to sit with your back to the door, and constantly scan the room."[118] The probability that patients will report traumatic symptoms that they have not in fact experienced is especially high when compensation is involved. Unlike other mental illnesses, a PTSD diagnosis can be a resource that entitles its bearers to obtain monetary and other benefits.[119]

Some observers claim that rising rates of PTSD among veterans are a product of a system that *promotes* disability. In an assertion that would not surprise World War I doctors and psychiatrists, a comprehensive review of the literature concluded in 2000 that "the specter of available disability benefits does influence the way in which veterans describe their difficulties, leading them to exaggerate symptoms either consciously or unconsciously."[120] The resulting benefits can be substantial. In 2014, successful claimants with 100 percent disability received an annual tax-free income of $34,884 if they were single and $39,216 if they were married and had two children, aside from any other resources available to them.[121] The latter is roughly the equivalent of the median income of families in half the states in the United States. Moreover, many of the recipients are mired in the income stagnation of working-class men who lack college degrees and have poor labor market prospects; this group would most benefit from the resources that a PTSD diagnosis secures. Financial need appears to be a major reason for the dramatic increase in recent rates of compensation-seeking for PTSD among veterans.[122]

In addition, the amount of compensation claimants obtain depends on their degree of impairment. For example, a veteran with no dependents receives a monthly payment of $133 for 10 percent disability but $2,907 for 100 percent disability. This creates a strong incentive to report as much impairment as possible. "Most veterans' self-reported symptoms of PTSD become worse over time until they reach 100 percent disability, at which point an 82 percent decline in use of VA mental health services occur," psychologist Christopher Frueh and colleagues report.[123] The systematic incentives to remain disabled in order to maintain benefits leads nearly all diagnosed veterans to report chronic conditions. One report indicates that "of the 572,612 veterans on the disability rolls for PTSD at the end of 2012, 1,868—a third of 1 percent—saw a reduction in their ratings the next year, according to statistics provided by the VA."[124] Psychiatrist Nancy Andreasen observes that VA policies are "problematic, in the sense that they require the person given compensation to be unemployed. This is a disincentive for full or even partial recovery."[125]

One study of veterans who were treated for chronic PTSD in a VA program, most of whom were Vietnam veterans, found that over half clearly exaggerated their symptoms.[126] Another archival study of help-seeking for PTSD among 100 Vietnam veterans during the late 1990s could verify that only 41 percent had been exposed to combat in Vietnam; 20 percent had served in Vietnam without evidence of combat exposure; 32 percent had served in Vietnam but did not appear to have seen combat; and the remaining 5 percent made false claims of service in Vietnam or even of any military service.[127] However, veterans who did not face combat applied for benefits at the same rate as those who did. Moreover, compensation-seeking veterans were more prone to over-report and exaggerate their symptoms and their service records than veterans who were not seeking compensation.[128] Nevertheless, almost all claimants received a PTSD diagnosis.

In sharp contrast to the eras in which previous wars were fought, there is little concern today that receiving compensation for PTSD promotes chronicity, prevents recovery, or threatens government finances. In 2007, an Institute of Medicine report observed that between 1999 and 2004, benefit payments for PTSD increased nearly 150 percent, from $1.72 billion to $4.28 billion.[129] In 2010 the VA dropped its requirement that veterans had to document battlefield events that caused trauma and expanded situations that could qualify to include fear of being attacked, regardless of whether any actual violence occurred. After the changes, the number of new PTSD claims rose 60 percent and approval rates jumped from 55 to 74 percent.[130]

A bipartisan consensus now exists for compensating disabled veterans with psychic damage. One congressman's explanation summarizes current political attitudes toward PTSD: "You don't have to prove it! You served us!"[131] The absence of stigma for PTSD diagnoses has removed one powerful barrier that prevented compensation-seeking in the past.

The lack of debate over whether PTSD diagnoses are always legitimate thoroughly contrasts with prior eras, when traumatic psychic injuries were regarded as easily simulated and traumatic diagnoses were seen as a good way to perpetuate, rather than cure, these conditions. Earlier observers would not be surprised at Erin Finley's observation: "If there is any one issue most likely to upset some visible minority of . . . frustrated veterans, it is the idea of *not* having PTSD. There are a variety of complex reasons for this, but one of the most important can be summed up in a single word: compensation."[132]

CONCLUSION

In certain respects, the expansion of post-traumatic stress disorder since the 1980s is just one illustration of the growing number of conditions that are viewed as mental illnesses. Rates of depression and anxiety, for example, have also exploded in recent decades.[133] The sources of the rise of therapeutic culture that Philip Rieff identified in the 1960s—the decline of communal values, more isolation of individuals, greater acceptability of viewing selves as vulnerable, lowered stigma for mental illness, and higher reliance on mental health professionals—are no different for PTSD than for other psychiatric conditions. In addition, various professional organizations, lay advocacy groups, and the research community have stimulated the increase in incidence of all forms of mental illness, including PTSD.

Nonetheless, the compassion for suffering that marks therapeutic cultures has probably influenced PTSD to a greater extent than any other mental illness. In particular, therapeutic cultures reject the possibility of malingering and other ways of taking advantage of mental illness labels, which are far more relevant to PTSD than to other conditions. Because it intrinsically involves some external entity that leads to emotional pain, PTSD raises issues of liability that are not present for other psychic impairments. It is uniquely suitable for obtaining compensation, particularly for veterans, who are an especially revered group. As Willard Waller noted after World War I, "He has fought for the flag and absorbed some of the *mana*. He is sacred. He is covered with pathos and immune from criticism."[134] While therapeutic cultures have enlarged the footprint of many forms of mental illness, they have particularly stimulated claims of PTSD.

Most observers regard the recent rise of therapeutic culture and the accompanying increase in PTSD diagnoses as signs of progress. What anthropologist Didier Fassin and political scientist Richard Rechtman call "the empire of trauma" is a moral revolution that has spawned a vast network of therapeutic interventions and accompanying rewards.[135] Clinicians herald the dramatic shift from the values of previous eras, which questioned the validity of claims of trauma victimization, to those that view traumatized people with sympathy and encourage them to seek mental health treatment. They especially appreciate the transformation in the cultural meanings attached to traumatic symptoms from the belief that many problems—especially those of traumatized men—that were formerly viewed as weakness of will or cowardice are in fact mental illnesses. Consequently, the stigma attached to a PTSD diagnosis has virtually disappeared, as has the belief that sufferers are responsible for their conditions. Disability benefits and other forms of compensation are far more readily available now than in the past. From this point of view, the major remaining problem is the incomplete penetration of therapeutic attitudes among resistant victims and social institutions.

Certain risks accompany the many positive aspects of the therapeutic mentality. Cultures can promote too much, as well as too little, remembrance of past traumas. As commentators over the past century and a half have noted, the benefits from a traumatic diagnosis can stabilize and prolong, rather than cure, conditions that might otherwise gradually dissipate on their own. A value system that stresses how traumatized people will have persistent psychic consequences unless they remain in treatment can become a self-fulfilling prophecy. Philip Rieff's son, the writer David Rieff, echoing the protagonist of *The Man in the Gray Flannel Suit*, notes how forgetting can be more therapeutic than remembering, "so that life can go on."[136] Expectations of inevitable, long-standing suffering and consequent rewards might underlie an unknown proportion of the current unprecedented levels of chronic PTSD.

Implications

When war conditions ceased to operate, the greater number
of the neurotic disturbances brought about by the war
simultaneously vanished.

Sigmund Freud, "Four Prefaces: Psychoanalysis and War Neuroses"

There is probably little we could now teach either the Regimental
Medical Officers of the First World War, or the psychiatrists of
the Second, about the psychological effects of war.

Simon Wessely, "Victimhood and Resilience"

The current acceptance of post-traumatic stress disorder as a legitimate psychiatric diagnosis thoroughly contrasts with its contentious history. The basic idea behind this stressor-related condition—that some traumatic event in the environment can lead
to lasting psychopathological consequences in previously normal
people—traditionally struggled to overcome psychiatric and cultural assumptions that mental disorders arise and persist because
of individual vulnerabilities or secondary rewards. As a result, the
evolution of PTSD involved constant tensions between, on the
one hand, the notion that external events traumatize blameless

victims, and, on the other hand, the focus on personal susceptibilities or suspicions of malingering.

The transformation of PTSD from a controversial and often disreputable condition to a widely recognized and credible diagnosis has broader implications for the study of psychiatric disorders. The combative history of PTSD helps to illuminate general issues about mental illnesses, including how they are defined, the extent to which they are viewed as products of internal or external forces, the conditions under which they are stigmatized or valued, the relationship between their biological and interpretative aspects, and how cultural values and social interests shape their nature.

DEFINING MENTAL DISORDERS

Like all mental disorders in the *DSM-5* (2013), the current definition of PTSD entails highly specific criteria. These include exposure to some severe stressor, intrusive memories of the traumatic event, persistent efforts to avoid recalling these distressing memories, impairing consequences that follow from recollections of the event, and hyperarousal connected with reminders of it.[1] This characterization follows from the general principle of psychiatric classification that arose in the *DSM-III* (1980), which dictated that all mental illnesses must have explicit, symptom-based definitions that are distinct from other clinical conditions. "Diagnosis, prognosis and treatment," historian Charles Rosenberg emphasizes, "have been linked ever more tightly to specific, agreed-upon disease categories."[2] Such precise descriptions provide a common ground to insure that different clinicians and researchers will recognize the same entities in their patients and research subjects. The current depiction of PTSD as a memory-related condition thus conforms to medical norms that dictate that legitimate diseases must be well-defined entities. It also distinguishes PTSD from diagnoses such as depression, anxiety, or psychosomatic conditions.

This portrayal of PTSD thoroughly contrasts with conceptualizations of stress-related disorders before the *DSM-III* revolution.

When trauma-related symptoms first arose during the nineteenth and early twentieth centuries, they were not differentiated from indicators of other common diagnoses, for example, hysteria or neurasthenia. The former featured a wide array of symptoms—emotional outbursts, fits, tics, tremors, fainting, and paralysis of limbs; the latter involved an even more capacious collection—depression, anxiety, fatigue, headaches, insomnia, overall weakness, and other indicators. Later, medical personnel during and after World War II emphasized how external shocks created an extensive variety of anxious, depressive, gastrointestinal, and psychosomatic consequences, which they called "combat neuroses" or "gross stress reactions." The broad term "physioneuroses," which involved general physiological, psychological, and social readjustments, also arose to characterize post-traumatic symptoms.

The conception of PTSD as a distinct memory-related syndrome resulting from exposure to trauma—rather than a generalized syndrome that is highly interrelated with other diagnostic conditions—stems more from the demands of professional norms than from congruence with any natural entity.[3] The *DSM* criteria that it exemplifies emerged because the psychiatric profession required a classification system that legitimated its status as physicians, provided it with the cultural prestige that accrues to those who combat genuine diseases, and allowed it to obtain reimbursement from insurers who demanded that clinicians treat specific entities.[4] The PTSD diagnosis itself resulted from a moral crusade by veterans who needed a condition that would both conform to *DSM* requirements and connect their psychic damage to external traumas that had occurred many years earlier. The remaking of PTSD from earlier depictions, which involved a range of bodily, emotional, and relational impacts to a specific disturbance of memory, provides a particularly powerful illustration of how social factors connected to professional and cultural legitimacy shape the nature of psychiatric diagnoses.

The current definition of PTSD is highly suitable for a number of groups. It provides trauma victims with a diagnosis that offers them an explanation for their psychic problems, moral vindication, therapy, and, in some cases, a reason to obtain compensation. It gives clinicians a way to be reimbursed for treating those who suffered traumas in the recent or the distant past. It offers researchers the precise criteria they need to know they are studying the same entity that other researchers are studying. Yet, the *DSM* definitions that have been institutionalized between 1980 and the present have severed PTSD from traditional understandings that stress-related conditions were interlocked with many forms of psychic suffering rather than specifically linked to traumatic memories. Professional demands about the nature of valid diseases led to the abandonment of the historical recognition that traumatic events produce a broad potpourri of psychological, bodily, and social consequences that cannot be pigeonholed into the categories of the *DSM*. A dramatic change in professional norms, not in the underlying nature of stressor-related conditions, accounts for current characterizations of PTSD.

EXTERNAL AND INTERNAL CAUSES OF MENTAL ILLNESS

The historical study of PTSD not only illuminates how social factors shape definitions of mental illness but also provides a valuable lens for viewing the vicissitudes of psychiatric explanations for why mental illnesses arise. The history of psychiatry has involved a perennial conflict between two divergent strains of thought. One view has emphasized the internal biological or psychological roots of mental illness, the other how external forces produce mental disturbances. The first position grounds mental disorders in flawed brains or nerves, which stem from physical defects or emotional weaknesses. When the psychiatric profession came into being in the nineteenth century, it focused on the presumably biological, and often inherited, roots of mental illness. Its organic and hereditarian assumptions could not easily encompass a diagnosis that associated stressful environments with lasting psychopathological consequences in previously normal people.

Following prevailing views at the time, the major initial students of trauma showed more interest in the presumed individual defects underlying traumatic conditions than in how external shocks produced mental disturbances. For example, Jean-Martin Charcot recognized that stressors caused by industrial accidents and train crashes produced a variety of hysterical symptoms.[5] He and other psychiatrists and neurologists, however, regarded external traumas as triggers, rather than causes, of mental pathology in predisposed victims. They were primarily concerned with the inherited factors that led some individuals who experienced these shocks, but not others, to develop hysteria. Charcot's student Pierre Janet examined how subconscious memories of a variety of stressors, including sickness, observing deaths, or viewing a variety of unpleasant stimuli during childhood could elicit traumas. Like Charcot, Janet viewed these stressors as provoking hysteria in previously susceptible patients.

Sigmund Freud revolutionized the study of traumatic stressors by providing a striking and unambiguous thesis: all cases of hysterical neuroses resulted from repressed memories of external sexual stimulation in infancy and childhood.[6] Although Freud challenged the dominant focus on heredity predispositions, he quickly repudiated his original view that actual traumatic sexual abuse during infancy and childhood produced hysteria. While he did not abandon the sexual etiology of traumatic symptoms, Freud came to believe that hysterical conditions arose from memories that were grounded in unconscious fantasies, not in real events. Nineteenth-century psychiatry thus remained thoroughly rooted in the internal foundations of mental disturbances.

The initial idea of purely stressor-related mental disorders developed outside of psychiatry. Well-publicized train crashes, in particular, appeared to create psychic damage among people who happened to be in the wrong place at the wrong time, not just among those who were already vulnerable to developing mental disorders.[7] Many people could empathize with the plights of the random victims of railroad crashes and industrial mishaps. Several decades later, the unprecedented slaughter of World War I led many psychiatrists, including Freud, to recognize that contemporaneous external traumas could produce psychic disturbances in anyone who was exposed to them, not just in the predisposed.[8]

Many physicians and psychiatrists, however, challenged assertions about the powerful pathological impacts of external shocks. This group highlighted how only some exposed people, but not others, became neurotic after even severe stressors. They also emphasized how shell shock was less likely to afflict soldiers who participated in battle than those who were nowhere near actual shelling or other forms of warfare but who feared going into battle. For example, a number of Freud's followers, underscoring how only a minority of soldiers exposed to combat developed mental illnesses, insisted that extreme stressors would only create impairments in people who were already prone to neuroses. Prominent psychoanalyst Karl Abraham claimed: "It is found with great regularity that war neurotics were even before the trauma . . . emotionally unstable, especially with regard to their sexuality."[9] One British study found that three-quarters of war-related psychological casualties had backgrounds marked by neuroses or psychoses compared to just 10 percent of a control group.[10] This outlook maintained the earlier focus on the internal vulnerabilities or character weaknesses that led to psychic collapse as opposed to the shocks from traumatic events themselves.

Some physicians at the time associated shell shock with individual predispositions, others with cowardice and malingering. Frederick Mott, a prominent British physician, stated the dominant opinion that most soldiers who suffered from a war neurosis possessed "an inborn timidity or neuropathic disposition, or an inborn germinal or acquired neuropathic or psychopathic taint."[11] Deeply rooted gender norms reinforced the contention that only cowards or men with other preexisting impairments would break down psychologically when anticipating or participating in combat. Even the carnage of World War I could not overturn the bedrock assumption among most medical personnel that normal men would not succumb to shell shock and other war-related neuroses.

The widespread medical acceptance of external traumas as sufficient causes of mental illness only appeared during the latter stages of World War II. Over the course of this war the previous emphasis on individual susceptibilities shifted to the view that stress-related symptoms were normal results of abnormal environments. By the end of the war, military psychiatrists agreed that "even the healthiest of individuals could break down under the influence of environmental stress."[12] Nonetheless, they still assumed that traumatic psychic consequences would be short-lived unless accompanied by internal predispositions. The psychiatric manuals that emerged after this war contained stressor-related disorders but only applied them to acute mental states. They assumed that some previously existing vulnerabilities or rewards from maintaining an impaired state accounted for pathology that persisted long after the initial stressor had ended. Thus, even after psychiatrists had accepted the legitimacy of stressor-related disorders, they continued to associate long-term or long-delayed conditions with individual susceptibilities rather than traumatic events.

An unequivocally stressor-related diagnosis only arose in 1980, as a result of strenuous lobbying efforts by Vietnam veterans and their advocates. The PTSD criteria in the *DSM-III* defined traumas as "outside the range of usual human experience" and rooted chronic or long-delayed, as well as brief, stress responses in the "existence of a recognizable stressor that would evoke significant symptoms of distress in almost everyone."[13] These were limited to occurrences such as military combat, rape, assault, and natural or man-made disasters. By clearly grounding symptoms in severe traumatic events, the diagnosis guaranteed the credibility of victims and ruled out the need to examine any preexisting biological or psychological vulnerabilities that made individuals prone to develop mental illness. It also dispensed with the consideration of character weaknesses, cowardice in particular, in accounting for mental breakdowns. One of the most prominent psychiatrists allied with the veterans, Chaim Shatan, emphasized the purely external nature of the *DSM-III* diagnosis: "After such massive man-made stress preexisting disorder is irrelevant. The specific stress itself constitutes the crucial predisposition."[14]

This exclusively exterior definition, however, created a problem that does not exist for other *DSM* conditions. Unlike other mental illnesses, the presence of symptoms alone cannot meet PTSD diagnostic criteria in the absence of an event that falls under the definition for what a "trauma" is. Therefore, uncertainties in PTSD diagnoses emerge over both what sorts of events qualify as "traumatic" and what are the most appropriate depictions of symptoms.

The fate of the *DSM-III* definition of trauma indicates how problematic psychiatry finds an unequivocally externally oriented mental illness. As in the past, many observers noted that not all persons exposed to even extreme stressors develop PTSD and that some individuals develop PTSD after even a minor stressor. Therefore, they emphasized, individual vulnerabilities must play some role in explaining this condition.[15] In response—in contrast to most of the manual's diagnoses, which have remained intact or undergone only minor changes through the present—the stressor criterion for PTSD continuously changed in revised editions of the *DSM*.

Subsequent manuals incorporated factors related to individual predispositions into the definition of what a "trauma" was: "the person's response involved intense fear, helplessness, or horror."[16] The inclusion of subjective responses in the diagnostic criteria extended the possible range of events considered to be "stressors" to encompass an ever-growing class of phenomena: worrisome election results, hearing objectionable speech, reading about violent actions, etc. Even people who did not directly experience a stressor but who were told about the death of a relative or watched a disaster unfold on television could suffer from a "trauma." The more expansive and subjective the criteria are for what defines a "stressor," the greater the likelihood that predispositions will have causal significance.[17]

The extensive revisions of the *DSM* criteria since 1980 echo the continuing uncertainties over the nature of traumatic diagnoses. Despite the initial grounding of the PTSD diagnosis in the impact of extreme stressors on previously normal individuals, the idea that personal vulnerabilities are an intrinsic aspect of all mental illnesses continues to resurface. Charcot or most World War I medical personnel could have written psychologist Marilyn Bowman and neuroscientist Rachel Yehuda's assertion that "PTSD is best understood as the periodic expression of long-standing dispositions that often are risk factors for both threatening exposures and subsequent dysfunctions."[18] Traumatologists are far from resolving issues about the extent to which stressors themselves or individual vulnerabilities to them account for who develops PTSD, what constitutes an event that is potentially traumatic, and the role of subjective interpretations in making a specific event "traumatic." The relationship between actual traumas and individual responses to them remains as problematic at present as it was when traumatic diagnoses were first developed.

THE DESIRABILITY OF MENTAL ILLNESS DIAGNOSES

PTSD not only provides insights into how definitions of and explanations for mental illnesses fluctuate over time but also illuminates some central aspects of responses to mental disturbances. Most labels of mental illness are associated with stigma, shame, and other undesirable consequences. They are typically negative assessments that people want to avoid, if possible. In contrast, PTSD, to an unusual extent among psychiatric diagnoses, can have favorable consequences. A British commission that investigated the implications of shell shock after World War I highlighted this aspect of stress-related diagnoses: "This class of case excited more general interest, attention, and sympathy than any other, so much so that it became a most desirable complaint from which to suffer."[19] Psychiatrist Nancy Andreasen's more recent observation echoes that report: "It is rare to find a psychiatric diagnosis that anyone likes to have, but PTSD seems to be one of them."[20] What accounts for the positive aspects of PTSD diagnoses, which so markedly differ from most psychiatric conditions?[21]

Unlike criteria for other mental illnesses, PTSD entails a causal connection between symptoms and some entity that can potentially be held liable for their emergence and persistence. When a public or private third party is responsible for a traumatic event and resultant suffering, victims gain not only an elevated moral status but, sometimes, financial rewards as well.[22] Before the purely stressor-related diagnosis emerged in the *DSM-III*, however, the worthiness of PTSD sufferers was highly contested. Because the damages of PTSD are internal, they are impossible to verify; self-reports provide the only evidence of traumatic psychic wounds. Coupled with the singular benefits of a PTSD diagnosis, the unconfirmable aspect of its symptoms traditionally led to deep suspicions over claims of enduring traumatic memories. While some clinicians have always argued that trauma victims deserve sympathy and help, others have viewed them with skepticism and scorn. The potential advantages from receiving a stressor-related diagnosis led to an association between PTSD and patient simulation to a possibly unique extent among mental illnesses.

From their inception, stressor-related conditions were deeply embedded in moral, as well as medical, contentions. PTSD only became a consequential form of mental illness when trauma victims could hold a specific party responsible for providing damages. "Railway spine," in particular, brought to the fore issues of compensation that have persisted throughout the history of PTSD. The widely publicized shocks of railway and other mechanized accidents could be tied to a well-defined and wealthy entity that could compensate the injured, including those with psychic wounds. Recall the observation of one British physician in 1866, who stated that the difference between a man being hurt in a railway accident and being hurt by falling out of a tree was that, "worse luck for him," he was not able to bring action against the tree.[23]

At the same time, allegations of psychological disability were vigorously countered by assertions that claimants were malingerers who sought to exploit the deep pockets of the railroads.[24] Nineteenth-century physicians who testified on behalf of railway companies emphasized how crash victims could easily fabricate psychological impairments that had no visible signs. Most juries in both Europe and the United States, however, rejected this argument and provided damages to those who brought lawsuits for their invisible psychic injuries.[25] This contentious framework persisted through World War I, when many physicians, citing the fact that many shell-shocked soldiers were not near the front lines of battle, raised the possibility that their traumatic symptoms arose as conscious or unconscious ways to escape combat. Officers, too, generally viewed mentally disabled soldiers as shirking their duties and simulating psychic injuries.[26]

Issues of PTSD and subsequent liability have been especially consequential when they involve government compensation and pensions.[27] Once national governments assumed responsibility for compensating psychologically impaired individuals, PTSD diagnoses became thoroughly entangled with socially defined issues of accountability, guilt, and damages. While these issues arose during the post–Civil War period, they became particularly acute in the post–World War I era, when the sheer number of claimants, coupled with the perilous economic circumstances of governments, rendered states wary of supporting such a large group of petitioners.[28] For most of the history of PTSD, governments were highly skeptical of claims of stress-related mental disabilities. For example, a British committee formed in 1939 to investigate the problem of pensions for shell-shocked veterans concluded: "There can be no doubt that in the overwhelming proportion of cases, these patients succumb to 'shock' because they get something out of it. To give them this reward is not ultimately a benefit to them because it encourages the weaker tendencies in their character."[29]

The initial medical and psychiatric assumptions about the nature of stress-related conditions bolstered the distrust of governments over the validity of disability claims for them. Even clinicians who did not question the reality of post-traumatic symptoms assumed that few cases would become chronic. Instead, they expected that extremely unpleasant traumatic states would naturally diminish in intensity with the passage of time and improving circumstances. Freud, for example, doubted the lingering impact of war trauma: "When war conditions ceased to operate, the greater number of the neurotic disturbances brought about by

the war simultaneously vanished."[30] Abram Kardiner, too, refer-
ring to the victims of an Italian earthquake, observed that "most
recovered within a few weeks, almost none remaining after six
months."[31] Most clinicians assumed that time-limited techniques,
which provided "an atmosphere of rest and assurance," would lead
most psychic injuries to heal fairly quickly.[32]

Many observers, however, singled out one striking exception
to the tendency for traumatic states to naturally dissipate over
short periods of time: the provision of compensation. In 1908, Édouard Brissaud, a student of Charcot's, noted that "in all the countries which provide compensation for accidents at work, 'insured'
injuries take much longer to heal than 'non-insured' injuries."[33]
During World War I, a Belgian observer warned: "It is time for us
to revise our ideas about traumatic neurosis and shell-shock. . . . If
we are not careful, if we do not plan correctly, we will see a legion
of false war invalids." He went to argue that there was "another,
rapid and radical, way of curing neurosis: refusing any compensation to the patient."[34] A German survey in 1925 went even further,
noting that "without the existence of liability laws of any kind,
accident or other avaricious pension neuroses would entirely not
exist."[35] Kardiner, too, was extremely sensitive to the role of compensation in facilitating lasting conditions: "On the basis of what
we know . . . about the traumatic neuroses, we can pose the question of whether this neurosis should be compensated. The answer
is decidedly that it should not."[36]

The issue of governmental accountability for stress-related
psychic wounds reemerged during the 1970s, when Vietnam veterans attributed their conditions to the immoral actions of the US
government and sought symbolic and material recompense from
it. The creation of the PTSD diagnosis in the *DSM-III* provided
a condition that allowed veterans to receive moral vindication,
treatment, and compensation without questioning their motiva-
tions.[37] Little consideration was given to the possibility, widely
recognized in previous eras, that telling individuals that they have
a persistent "post-traumatic stress disorder" can send a message
that their emotions are pathologies in need of lengthy treatments

instead of normal responses to extremely stressful environments. This message might unwittingly divert attention from natural tendencies to resilience and self-healing and stabilize symptoms that could otherwise dissipate with time.[38]

Perhaps more important, providing monetary compensation to PTSD sufferers might provide an *inducement* to maintain chronic conditions. In the past, clinicians would have been especially wary of compensating stressor-related conditions that did not emerge immediately after the trauma but only became apparent years, or even decades, afterward. The most common attitude toward these delayed conditions was that of an American pension board, which ruled that a Civil War veteran's family was not entitled to payment: "Rejection, on the ground that soldier's death from suicide in 1875 can in no way be attributed to his military service from which he was discharged in 1865."[39] Its assumption was that any psychic consequences would become manifest at the time of the traumatic event, not at a much later period. Traumas would have immediate impacts that should gradually dissipate, not intensify, over time.

Issues regarding long-dormant symptoms became especially prominent in the 1970s, when many Vietnam veterans demanded recognition of conditions that had been latent for many years: "Many veterans did not react immediately to this stress and only became 'psychiatric casualties' months and even years after their return to the United States."[40] Indeed, PTSD claims among this group in particular soared in the early twenty-first century, decades after the cessation of combat. In contrast to the situation in earlier eras, a long lapse between the event and its psychic consequences no longer discredited disability claims. For the first time in its history, PTSD came to be viewed as a chronic condition that did not diminish in strength with the passage of time. Successful claims are especially easy to make when petitioners are not stigmatized, and their claims are not closely examined.[41]

It is difficult to explain the enormous rise since the millennium in PTSD petitions from survivors of long-past wars without considering the advantages that accrue from this diagnosis.[42] In particular, the emergence of a huge epidemic of PTSD so many years after the Vietnam War ended is hard to reconcile with a substantial literature that indicates traumatic memories gradually lose their forcefulness.[43] Current disability programs, which cut benefits when patients no longer report traumatic symptoms, can actively *promote* chronicity by punishing those who improve and rewarding those who maintain enduring conditions. Remarkably, as the previous chapter noted, more than 99 percent of veterans receiving disability payments for PTSD from the Veterans Administration do not improve in the following year.[44] As psychiatrists traditionally recognized, systemic reinforcements encourage enduring states of post-traumatic disability. In the case of PTSD, the compassion and caring that marks the therapeutic mentality might facilitate lifelong disability instead of recovery.[45] "America's war veterans, who are entitled to our respect and support," psychiatrist Paul McHugh observes, "certainly deserve better than to be maintained in a state of chronic invalidism."[46]

BIOLOGY AND INTERPRETATION

The history of PTSD also helps shed light on how both biological and interpretive factors shape the nature of mental disorders. Since the emergence of psychiatry in the nineteenth century, "real" disorders were those with some grounding in the brain.[47] Stressor-related conditions challenged this bedrock tenet because it appeared that some purely psychic process connected memories of a past traumatic event with the subsequent emergence of symptoms. Issues regarding the relative importance of physical and psychological influences have been perennial aspects in the debate over the nature of PTSD.

Brains and Minds

The initial discussions about the importance of organic and psychic features of traumatic symptoms involved the extent to which the impact of railway and other accidents worked through neural or mental routes. One perspective—exemplified in the work of John Erichsen and Hermann Oppenheim—assumed that powerful external stressors created actual neurological changes that, in turn, resulted in psychic symptoms. A second strand of thought—represented by Jean-Martin Charcot, Pierre Janet, and Sigmund Freud—emphasized the mental pathways that linked traumas to psychological disturbances. By the end of the nineteenth century two distinct schools had developed, one arguing that psychic injuries that arose after traumas were organically based and the other that they were psychological in nature.[48] The same contention reemerged during World War I, as some medical observers insisted that wartime traumas led to actual brain damages, while others associated them with purely psychic fear and terror.

Psychiatry's environmental turn, which began during World War II and continued through the mid-1970s, left no room for the biological aspects of PTSD. When brain-based frameworks reemerged at this time, they came with a vengeance. Widespread sentiment arose—in many ways echoing prevailing nineteenth-century views—that PTSD must be connected to some brain-based defect. In particular, the emergence of neuroscience as a dominant force in psychiatry and psychology reenergized the search for the biological correlates of PTSD. Armed with the powerful tools of fMRI and other imaging technologies, neuroscientists set out to discover the visible damages that traumas afflict on the brain.

Many researchers, clinicians, and funding agencies have turned to neuroscience as the best hope for making future advancements in defining and treating PTSD (as well as other mental disorders). A seemingly boundless optimism characterizes much neuroscientific writing regarding PTSD. In 2001 Nancy Andreasen predicted: "Our questions about the nature and role of unconscious memories, forgotten memories, false memories, flashbulb memories, and intrusive unwanted memories will probably all be explained during the next several decades, as we understand more and more about how the hippocampus and amygdala work with one another and with other sites distributed throughout the brain."[49] The enthusiasm surrounding neuroscience has also made its way into popular culture, where phrases such as "stress damages the brain," or the brains of PTSD sufferers have been "permanently changed," have become commonplace.[50]

A growing number of studies attempts to identify the neurobiological correlates of PTSD in order to provide a diagnostic marker for this condition. In accord with nineteenth-century neurologists and psychiatrists, neuroscientists believe that uncovering a biological indicator will legitimate traumatic disorders as genuine diseases. A brain-based substrate would, according to neuroscientists Rachel Yehuda and Alexander McFarlane, provide "an essential first step in allowing the permanent validation of human suffering."[51] In the 2015 epilogue to her canonical book, *Trauma and Recovery*, Judith Herman asserts that neuroimaging techniques can even reveal the specific regions of the brain where unconscious traumatic memories reside: "Advances in neurobiology have documented the effects of trauma on the brain that cause 'repressed memories.'"[52] It is possible, however, that uncovering the specific brain correlates that identify PTSD would *limit* the pool of legitimate sufferers who can obtain a diagnosis by disqualifying traumatized people who do not show the appropriate biological damage.

Despite the confidence of many neuroscientists that they will soon discover the biological basis of post-traumatic stress disorder, central questions remained unanswered. To date, all efforts to find biological indicators that make people prone to develop PTSD have failed.[53] In 2006 an Institute of Medicine report concluded that "no biomarkers are clinically useful or specific in diagnosing PTSD, assessing the risk of developing it, or charting its progression."[54] Moreover, such neural signatures might not be unique to PTSD but instead be connected to more general vulnerabilities that are also present in anxiety and depression, for example. Little evidence shows that the biological aspects of PTSD are *uniquely* associated with the consequences of exposure to external shocks.[55] Neuroscientists will also face the challenge of disentangling whether biological flaws are the result or the cause of PTSD. As Stephen Hyman, a former director of the National Institute of Mental Health (NIMH) notes, a gaping disconnect exists between the discoveries of molecular neuroscience and their translation into useful clinical responses.[56]

Achieving the long-standing aspiration to relate traumas with subsequent brain damage would undoubtedly assist in identifying and effectively treating PTSD sufferers. If they could be developed, drugs that target the specific brain regions where traumatic memories are located might eliminate their intrusive and distressing qualities.[57] Nevertheless, the emergence of precise drug interventions or brain-based diagnostic markers would not erase the need to consider the intrinsically *moral* aspects of stressor-related conditions. The PTSD diagnosis, as Didier Fassin and Richard Rechtman note, "identifies complaints as justified and causes as just."[58] Cultural values, not brain images, are the ultimate validators of traumatic suffering.

Universality and Relativity

The history of PTSD also helps illuminate the extent to which mental illnesses are universal and timeless or historical and culturally specific. This book grounded the initial emergence of stressor-related diagnoses in changes connected to nineteenth-century social life, culture, and professional ideology. Mechanized accidents stemmed from an entity that could be causally linked to—and held liable for—resultant symptoms. At the same time, new psychiatric conceptions of memory provided plausible explanations for continuing suffering after traumas.[59]

Much recent literature offers a starkly contrasting view. A number of psychiatrists, psychologists, and classicists, as well as some historians, argue that because the brains of current humans show few biological differences from those of our distant ancestors, the discovery of brain correlates of PTSD indicates its timeless qualities. For them, neuroscientific findings that uncover a biological signature of PTSD indicate that this condition must have been present, albeit unrecognized, throughout history. For example, historian Lawrence Tritle contends that PTSD has been a perpetual aspect of the human experience because of its "underlying human physiology, a constant for the last 200,000 years."[60]

The presumed universal aspects of PTSD have been used to diagnose with hindsight the responses to traumas among literary and historical figures such as Achilles, Odysseus, Socrates, Alexander the Great, Samuel Pepys, and Emily Dickinson.[61]

Ancient Greece has been the most common locus of retrospective diagnoses, almost always of combat-related reactions. The historical perspective taken here indicates that, although the Greeks had sophisticated medical understandings of disturbed behaviors, it would have been inconceivable for them to apply these conceptions to the psychic consequences of battle. The Greeks associated combat with issues concerning honorable and dishonorable conduct, not with any medical condition: "Ability to fight in close combat was the highest and most glorious expression of the masculine ideal."[62] Conversely, deep shame was attached to soldiers who could not uphold norms of courage and manliness. Cowards had deeply flawed character traits, not diseases; they became social outcasts who lost all rights as citizens.[63]

Greek brains might be similar to our own, but Greek interpretations of brain-based states did not resemble modern views of traumas and their consequences. The cultural preconditions for stressor-related diagnoses were not present until relatively recently. Even if neuroscientific studies were to find an unambiguous brain signature of what we call "PTSD," traumas would not have had the same psychic consequences before the nineteenth century as they do at present. PTSD, like all mental phenomena, might be partly biological, but it also consists of an irreducible cultural aspect.

The Cultural Symptom Pool

Another contribution that the historical study of PTSD makes is to provide a powerful example of how historically and culturally based templates structure the particular expressions of mental disorders. Historian Edward Shorter posits that symptoms of mental illnesses do not directly indicate brain states but instead stem from cultural models.[64] While the manifest symptoms of a few psychiatric conditions, such as dementia or syphilis, might reflect timeless aspects of brains, the overt expressions of most mental illnesses arise from what Shorter calls "the symptom pool." This term refers to whatever symptomatic presentations the general culture and the medical profession validate in any particular historical period. Sufferers unconsciously model their symptoms after illnesses that are popular at the time and that their doctors expect them to display. Once medical diagnostic fashions change, patients follow suit and develop the kinds of symptoms that the newest style promotes.

The power of culturally shaped symptom pools could explain the vast changes in the overt presentations of stressor-related conditions over time. For example, in 1871, before a psychological diagnosis was available, an army surgeon, Jacob Da Costa, coined the term "irritable heart syndrome" to describe the palpitations, cardiac pain, numbness of the arm, rapid pulse, shortness of breath, and sweating he observed among combat veterans of the American Civil War. Although Da Costa could not associate these symptoms with any physiological abnormalities in hearts, this organ provided a culturally acceptable basis for traumatic symptoms. Later, the horrific conditions of World War I led many soldiers to develop widely known symptoms associated with hysteria, such as paralysis of limbs, inability to speak, or blindness, despite having no apparent somatic pathology. The term "shellshock" entered the symptom pool so that physicians would not have to diagnose these men with the female-linked condition of hysteria. The mostly physiological symptoms connected with shell shock bore little resemblance to the depressive and anxious states that prevailed during World War II or to the presentations of PTSD among Vietnam veterans, who often reported flashbacks to traumatic combat-related experiences, expressions that were rare among combatants in previous wars.[65] Even if PTSD has a neurological basis, history shows that any biological substructure must have an interpretative superstructure that shapes the manifest presentations of the constantly changing symptoms of this condition.

Social Values and Interests

A striking aspect of the transformation of PTSD from a condition marked by weakness, suspicion, and conscious or unconscious malingering to a diagnosis that warrants compassion, sympathy, and reward is how little it had to do with developments within the psychiatric profession. Most illnesses, whether physical or mental, are grounded in what Charles Rosenberg describes as "a web of practice guidelines, disease protocols, laboratory and imaging results, meta-analyses, and consensus conferences."[66] In thoroughgoing contrast, the scientific study of PTSD in laboratories, fMRI machines, and epidemiological research *followed* rather than preceded its inclusion into the disease canon.[67]

The current PTSD diagnosis emerged as a result of the moral demands of lay victims for recognition of their suffering. It arose from the lobbying efforts of Vietnam veterans who sought justification, treatment, and compensation for their psychic wounds. Lay advocates had to overcome professional *resistance* to a diagnosis that established a causal link between wartime traumas and resulting symptoms.[68] Their objectives conflicted with the psychiatric profession's new classificatory system, which eschewed causal claims and viewed only specific, well-defined conditions that are distinct from other diagnoses as legitimate mental illnesses. Mental health professionals thoroughly embraced the PTSD diagnosis after it appeared in the *DSM-III*, but they were not responsible for its inclusion in this manual.

Another unusual aspect of PTSD is that the substantial establishment devoted to studying and treating trauma has largely developed independently of the psychiatric and other extant mental health professions. Instead, a new vocation of grief and trauma counselors, without historical predecessors, has become widely institutionalized in many educational, medical, governmental, and business entities. The condition has developed its own professional societies and journals, which are devoted to the study of trauma. The chief source of support for researchers who study

PTSD, the Veterans' Administration, is also distinct from the primary provider of funding for other mental illnesses, the NIMH. The major groups that publicize PTSD are victims' associations, private charities, and relief agencies.[69] PTSD not only originally emerged in response to lay demands, but it persists in public consciousness as a result of the efforts of a web of organizations, occupations, and activities that is largely separate from medical and psychiatric specialists.

PTSD is also distinctive among current prominent psychiatric diagnoses because of its independence from the pharmaceutical industry. The marketing efforts of drug companies have been extraordinarily influential in promoting other common mental illnesses—depression, anxiety, bipolar disorder, attention deficit disorder.[70] While clinicians prescribe a capacious potpourri of drugs, including antidepressants, antipsychotics, sedatives, mood stabilizers, amphetamines, and opioids, for PTSD patients, none of these drugs was developed for PTSD, none is advertised as a treatment for it, and none has proven to be very effective for dealing with it.[71] In contrast to their role with other mental disorders, drug companies have had a negligible part in shaping social responses to PTSD.

Lay efforts that led to the PTSD diagnosis—and the large trauma establishment that developed as a consequence—themselves reflect the assumptions and expectations of the culture of therapy that arose in the United States and other Western countries in the final decades of the twentieth century.[72] While the institutionalization of this culture enlarged the footprint of and provided unquestioned legitimacy to many forms of mental illness, it especially stimulated the growth of PTSD. The therapeutic viewpoint's particular attunement to the vulnerability of individuals to external stressors resonated with essential aspects of PTSD. Trauma culture broadened the definition of what constitutes a "trauma," expanded the pool of people who are prone to develop traumas, and called for sympathetic responses to those who were victims of traumatic conditions. Conversely, the tenets of this culture preclude assertions of malingering or other means of taking advantage of mental illness labels, which had limited the widespread recognition of PTSD in the past.

Therapeutic culture encompasses men as well as women, thus severing the link between masculinity and invulnerability to stressors that had persisted for centuries.[73] PTSD quickly spread through the general culture as an emblematic condition of the new therapeutic ethos among males and females alike. It is far more congruent with a social climate that is attuned to concerns with mental health and victimization than with traditional notions of courage and cowardice.[74]

The acceptance of PTSD as a genuine disease is consensually viewed as a welcome development for traumatized people. "It is widely taken for granted that the adoption of PTSD in DSM-III was unequivocally a good thing from a clinical point of view," anthropologist Allan Young and epidemiologist Naomi Breslau observed in 2007.[75] Current healing-oriented responses have replaced both the stoic attitudes that led the afflicted to bear their psychic wounds silently and the punitive responses to traumatized people that often prevailed in previous eras. Therapeutic values have destigmatized the recognition of and help-seeking for traumatic conditions and so have allowed multitudes of sufferers to receive mental health care. They have also largely silenced the perennial debates between those who viewed either exposure to traumatic events or vulnerability to these events as the central aspect of PTSD. Therapeutic culture views traumatic conditions that develop among both the exposed and the vulnerable as equally deserving of compassionate responses.

Therapeutic orientations have become so powerful that they have attained virtually universal acceptance. While such views existed in the past, they were always met with considerable opposition from military, political, and medical institutions. At present, however, no competing groups resist the therapeutic view of PTSD. Indeed, as the previous chapter noted, it is one of the rare conditions that bridges partisan positions. In addition, it also unites the bitter divides between liberal and conservative news media that have marked the initial year of the Trump presidency. For example, the extensive coverage of PTSD on Fox News and in the *New York Times* is virtually indistinguishable.[76] Each outlet portrays the struggles of veterans and others to cope with PTSD in a sympathetic light; neither raises issues of simulation or malingering. In the case of PTSD, all sides of the political spectrum embrace the tenets of therapy culture as an enlightened and welcome response to traumatized victims.

THE FUTURE OF PTSD

The current omnipresence of the PTSD diagnosis stems from its recognition of the profound psychic impact of traumatic injuries as well as its enabling of the means to seek therapeutic solutions for them. It provides explanations that help alleviate the suffering of victims, who have embraced its use. In this sense, therapeutic narratives represent progress over past accounts, which focused on cowardice, simulation, malingering, unconscious conflicts, and the like.[77]

Despite the cultural and professional acceptance of PTSD as a legitimate psychiatric disorder, we still have limited knowledge about the nature of trauma, why it has such variable impacts on different individuals, and, especially, how to most effectively treat it. Psychiatrist Simon Wessely tellingly observes that "there is probably little we could now teach either the Regimental Medical Officers of the First World War, or the psychiatrists of the Second, about the psychological effects of war."[78] The difficulties in defining and responding to PTSD that mental health professionals have faced through the earliest inception of traumatic diagnoses in the nineteenth century, the major wars of the twentieth and twenty-first centuries, and the recurring problems of sexual victimizations, terrorist attacks, and natural disasters are unlikely to be resolved in the foreseeable future.

Indeed, the historical study of stressor-related conditions reveals the flaws, as well as the advantages, of current definitions of them. When PTSD entered the *DSM-III* in 1980, legitimate psychiatric diagnoses were ones that possessed a core of well-defined symptoms. Since that time, however, many psychiatrists and other mental health professionals have become disillusioned over the lack of progress in understanding and treating mental disorders. A current of discontent with the categorical diagnoses of the whole array of mental disorders in the *DSM* has arisen that might have especially profound effects on PTSD. This sentiment is driving the Research Domain Criterion—a current initiative of the NIMH—which seeks to create a new dimensional taxonomy that includes behavioral as well as neurobiological measures.[79] New ways of conceiving of mental disorders, which in many respects resemble past characterizations, see them as interlocking rather than distinct, as incorporating psychological, cultural, social, and biological layers, and as involving contextual along with individualized treatments.[80]

While the future success of such efforts is unclear, their realization could be especially salutary for defining, explaining, and treating PTSD. The multifaceted results of traumas are not well-suited for a diagnostic system that requires highly specific and distinct syndromes. As many observers in prior eras recognized, the challenging readjustments that traumatic conditions require inherently occur within social, as well as psychological and biological, contexts. Horrific and shocking experiences uproot people's basic sense of values and reality and their fundamental assumptions regarding personal safety, mortality, and a just world. Such disturbing events often require the reconstruction of meaning systems to suit new circumstances. An overemphasis on recollecting traumatic memories can both deflect considerations of reintegration and prolong suffering that might otherwise gradually dissolve. The specificity of the current *DSM* diagnostic system—whatever value it might have for other psychiatric disorders—is particularly ill-suited for understanding PTSD and helping its victims.

NOTES

Chapter 1. A Disorder through Time

1. W. H. Auden, *The Age of Anxiety* (1947; Princeton, NJ: Princeton University Press, 2011); Allan V. Horwitz and Jerome C. Wakefield, *The Loss of Sadness: Psychiatry's Transformation of Normal Sadness into Depressive Disorder* (New York: Oxford University Press, 2007). Between 1990 and 2008 Google Ngram shows that the use of the term "PTSD" increased by about 350 percent. For a particularly good example of the expanding use of the term, see http://www.cbsnews.com/news/have-you-been-traumatized -by-2016/, retrieved September 17, 2017.

2. Mary Kerr, "Trump's Win Shows Us It's Time to Listen, but Not Forget," *New Yorker*, November 21, 2016, 59; Diane Jhueck, "A Clinical Case for the Dangerousness of Donald J. Trump," in *The Dangerous Case of Donald Trump*, ed. Bandy Lee (New York: St. Martin's Press, 2017), 181–197, 186.

3. American Psychiatric Association, *Diagnostic and Statistical Manual of Mental Disorders*, 3rd ed. (Washington, DC: American Psychiatric Association, 1980), 238.

4. Allan Young, *The Harmony of Illusions: Inventing Post-Traumatic Stress Disorder* (Princeton, NJ: Princeton University Press, 1995), 130.

5. The most prominent illustration was the prediction (which was not fulfilled) that huge numbers of people would suffer from PTSD and other mental disorders after the September 11, 2001, terrorist attacks. Melvin Konner, "Trauma, Adaptation, and Resilience: A Cross-Cultural and Evolutionary Perspective," in *Understanding Trauma*, ed. Lawrence Kirmayer, Robert Lemelson, and Mark Barad (New York: Cambridge University Press, 2007), 300–338, 313.

6. Alan Zerembo, "As Disability Awards Grow, So Do Concerns with Veracity of PTSD Claims," *Los Angeles Times*, August 3, 2014.

7. Richard J. McNally and B. Christopher Frueh, "Why Are Iraq and Afghanistan War Veterans Seeking PTSD Disability Compensation at Unprecedented Rates?," *Journal of Anxiety Disorders* 27 (2013): 520–526, 520.

8. Paul Lerner and Mark S. Micale, "Trauma, Psychiatry, and History: A Conceptual and Historiographical Introduction," in *Traumatic Pasts:*

History, Psychiatry, and Trauma in the Modern Age, 1870–1930, ed. Mark S. Micale and Paul Lerner (New York: Cambridge University Press, 2001), 3.

9. E.g., Michael MacDonald, *Mystical Bedlam: Madness, Anxiety, and Healing in Seventeenth-Century England* (New York: Cambridge University Press, 1981); Steven Pinker, *The Better Angels of Our Nature: Why Violence Has Declined* (New York: Penguin, 2012).

10. John Keegan, *The Face of Battle* (New York: Penguin, 1983), 319.

11. Young, *Harmony of Illusions,* 7.

12. Patrick McGrath, *Trauma: A Novel* (New York: Vintage, 2008), 131.

13. Erin P. Finley, *Fields of Combat* (Ithaca, NY: ILR Press, 2012), 59.

14. Judith Herman, *Trauma and Recovery: The Aftermath of Violence— From Domestic Abuse to Political Terror* (New York: Basic Books, 2015), 1.

15. Quoted in Mikkel Borch-Jacobsen, "Self-Seduced," in *Unauthorized Freud,* ed. Frederick Crews (New York: Penguin, 1998), 43–53, 50.

16. "Stress" is often used to refer to the cause of some set of symptoms. In PTSD, however, it refers to the *result* of some trauma.

17. Richard J. McNally, *Remembering Trauma* (Cambridge, MA: Harvard University Press, 2003), 9; Young, *Harmony of Illusions,* 7.

18. Paul R. McHugh, *Try to Remember: Psychiatry's Clash over Meaning, Memory, and Mind* (New York: Dana Press, 2008), 183.

19. Willard W. Waller, *The Veteran Comes Back* (1944; San Francisco: Forgotten Books, 2006), 166.

20. E.g., Naomi Breslau, Glenn C. Davis, Patricia Andreski, Belle Federman, and James C. Anthony, "Traumatic Events and Post-traumatic Stress Disorder in an Urban Population of Young Adults," *Archives of General Psychiatry* 48 (1991): 216–222.

21. See http://www.integration.samhsa.gov/clinical-practice/trauma, retrieved July 15, 2017.

22. Talcott Parsons, *The Social System* (Glencoe, IL: Free Press, 1951).

23. Chris Cantor, *Evolution and Posttraumatic Stress* (New York: Routledge, 2005); Susan Mineka, "Evolutionary Memories, Emotional Processing, and the Emotional Disorders," *Psychology of Learning and Motivation* 28 (1992): 161–206; Allan V. Horwitz and Jerome C. Wakefield, *All We Have to Fear: Psychiatry's Transformation of Natural Anxieties into Mental Disorders* (New York: Oxford University Press, 2012).

24. Gerald N. Grob and Allan V. Horwitz, *Diagnosis, Therapy, and Evidence* (New Brunswick, NJ: Rutgers University Press, 2010), 164.

25. Edward Shorter, *A History of Psychiatry: From the Era of Psychiatry to the Age of Prozac* (New York: John Wiley & Sons, 1997).

26. Charles Rycroft, *Anxiety and Neurosis* (London: Maresfield Library, 1968), 25.

27. Gerald N. Grob, *From Asylum to Community* (Princeton, NJ: Princeton University Press, 1991), 16.

28. Institute of Medicine, *Treatment of PTSD: An Assessment of the Evidence* (Washington, DC: National Academies Press, 2007).

29. E.g., Waller, *Veteran Comes Back*.

30. Nancy Andreasen, "Posttraumatic Stress Disorder: Psychology, Biology, and the Manichean Warfare between False Dichotomies," *American Journal of Psychiatry* 152 (1995): 964.

31. Ralph Harrington, "The Railway Accident: Trains, Trauma, and Technological Crises in Nineteenth-Century Britain," in Micale and Lerner, *Traumatic Pasts*, 31–56 (see n8); Eric Caplan. "Trains and Trauma in the American Gilded Age," in ibid., 57–77; Eric Caplan, "Trains, Brains, and Sprains: Railway Spine and the Origins of Psychoneuroses," *Bulletin of the History of Medicine* 69 (1995): 387–419.

32. Southborough, 1922, quoted in Edgar Jones and Simon Wessely, *Shell Shock to PTSD: Military Psychiatry from 1900 to the Gulf War* (New York: Psychology Press, 2005), 54, 151. This report concluded that shell shock should be "eliminated from official nomenclature" because well-trained troops would not develop shell shock. Edgar Jones, Ian Palmer, and Simon Wessely, "War Pensions (1900–1945): Changing Models of Psychological Understanding," *British Journal of Psychiatry* 180 (2002): 374–379, 376.

33. Parsons, *The Social System*.

34. John M. Kinder, *Paying with Their Bodies: American War and the Problem of the Disabled Veteran* (Chicago: University of Chicago Press, 2015), 164, 197.

35. E.g., Elaine Showalter, *Hystories: Hysterical Epidemics and Modern Culture* (New York: Columbia University Press, 1988).

36. E.g., David Finkel, *Thank You for Your Service* (New York: Farrar, Straus & Giroux, 2013).

37. Nancy Andreasen, *Brave New Brain: Conquering Mental Illness in the Era of the Genome* (New York: Oxford University Press, 2001).

38. For example, the first sentence of a major handbook about PTSD reads, "Throughout the history of mankind, traumatic events of natural and human origin have occurred that have left psychic scars on the inner selves of the victims and the survivors." John P. Wilson and Beverley Raphael, "Theoretical and Conceptual Foundations of Traumatic Stress Syndromes," in *International Handbook of Traumatic Stress Syndromes*, ed. J. P. Wilson and B. Raphael (New York: Plenum Press, 1993), 1–9, 1. Similarly, psychiatrist Michael Trimble's historical study of PTSD concludes that "this relatively common human problem has been known for many hundreds of years, although under different names." Michael R. Trimble, *Post-Traumatic Neu-*

rosis: From Railway Spine to the Whiplash (New York: John Wiley & Sons, 1981), 5.

39. Yulia Ustinova and Etzel Cardeña, "Combat Stress Disorders and Their Treatment in Ancient Greece," *Psychological Trauma: Theory, Research, Practice, and Policy* (2014), http://dx.doi.org/10.1037/a0036461), 1.

40. E.g., Young, *Harmony of Illusions*; Micale and Lerner, *Traumatic Pasts*; Ian Hacking, *The Social Construction of What?* (Cambridge, MA: Harvard University Press, 1999); Didier Fassin and Richard Rechtman, *The Empire of Trauma* (Princeton, NJ: Princeton University Press, 2009).

41. Hacking, *The Social Construction of What?*, 100.

42. McNally, *Remembering Trauma*, 283.

43. Henri F. Ellenberger, *The Discovery of the Unconscious: The History and Evolution of Dynamic Psychiatry* (New York: Basic Books, 1970), 749.

44. Georges Deveroux, *Basic Problems in Ethnopsychiatry* (Chicago: University of Chicago Press, 1980).

45. Mikkel Borch-Jacobsen, *Making Minds and Madness: From Hysteria to Depression* (New York: Cambridge University Press, 2009), 21–22.

46. Young, *Harmony of Illusions*, 5.

Chapter 2. PTSD Emerges

1. Around the same time, Europeans recognized the psychological consequences of the Franco-Prussian war of 1870–71. See Ian Hacking, *Rewriting the Soul* (Princeton, NJ: Princeton University Press, 1995), 188.

2. "Courage and Cowardice," *New York Times*, August 14, 1861.

3. Drew Gilpin Faust, *This Republic of Suffering: Death and the Civil War* (New York: Vintage, 2008), 41.

4. Faust, *This Republic of Suffering*, xi; John M. Kinder, *Paying with Their Bodies: American War and the Problem of the Disabled Veteran* (Chicago: University of Chicago Press, 2015), 22; Michael C. C. Adams, *Living Hell: The Dark Side of the Civil War* (Baltimore: Johns Hopkins University Press, 2014), 11.

5. Adams, *Living Hell*, 15; Faust, *This Republic of Suffering*, 32–33.

6. Eric T. Dean Jr., *Shook over Hell: Post-Traumatic Stress, Vietnam, and the Civil War* (Cambridge, MA: Harvard University Press, 1991), 121, 146.

7. Adams, *Living Hell*, 25; Frances Clarke, "So Lonesome I Could Die: Nostalgia and Debates over Emotional Control in the Civil War North," *Journal of Social History* 41 (Winter, 2007).

8. Dean, *Shook over Hell*, 131.

9. Brian M. Jordan, *Marching Home: Union Veterans and Their Unending Civil War* (New York: W. W. Norton, 2014), 128.

10. Dean, *Shook over Hell*, 120.

11. Faust, *This Republic of Suffering*, 5, 6.

12. Dean, *Shook over Hell*, 202.
13. Adams, *Living Hell*, 124, 128.
14. Adams, *Living Hell*, 110.
15. Jordan, *Marching Home*, 189.
16. Dean, *Shook over Hell*, 111.
17. Adams, *Living Hell*, 125.
18. Dean, *Shook over Hell*, 106.
19. Adams, *Living Hell*, 125.
20. Adams, *Living Hell*, 183.
21. Dean, *Shook over Hell*, 134.
22. Kinder, *Paying with Their Bodies*, 26.
23. Kinder, *Paying with Their Bodies*, 30.
24. Jordan, *Marching Home*, 33.
25. Jordan, *Marching Home*, 189.
26. Jordan, *Marching Home*, 185.
27. Andrew Scull, *Madness in Civilization* (Princeton, NJ: Princeton University Press, 2015), 274.
28. The American neurologist George Beard coined the medical diagnosis of "neurasthenia" in 1869 to refer to a general weakness of the nervous system marked by a wide array of symptoms, including fatigue, anxiety, depression, headache, impotence, and depression, among many others. It was most commonly, although not exclusively, applied to middle- and upper-class men. George M. Beard, *American Nervousness: Its Causes and Consequences* (New York: G. P. Putnam's Sons, 1881).
29. Jordan, *Marching Home*, 189.
30. Paul W. Skerritt, "Anxiety and the Heart—A Historical Review," *Psychological Medicine* 13 (1983): 17–25.
31. Paul Wood, "Da Costa's Syndrome," *British Medical Journal*, May 24, 1941, 805–811. During the nineteenth century, many British soldiers were discharged from duty because of heart conditions that physicians thought were a result of the heavy equipment they had carried. Edgar Jones and Simon Wessely, *Shell Shock to PTSD: Military Psychiatry from 1900 to the Gulf War* (New York: Psychology Press, 2005), 9.
32. Dean, *Shook over Hell*, 200.
33. Dean, *Shook over Hell*, 67.
34. Adams, *Living Hell*, 201.
35. Dean, *Shook over Hell*, 104.
36. Adams, *Living Hell*, 126.
37. Faust, *This Republic of Suffering*, 196.
38. Kinder, *Paying with Their Bodies*, 24.
39. Jordan, *Marching Home*, 70.
40. Adams, *Living Hell*, 108.

41. Kinder, *Paying with Their Bodies*, 3.

42. Kinder, *Paying with Their Bodies*, 26.

43. Dean, *Shook over Hell*, 144.

44. Dean, *Shook over Hell*, 148.

45. Dean, *Shook over Hell*, 147.

46. Jordan, *Marching Home*, 162.

47. Jordan, *Marching Home*, 167.

48. Kinder, *Paying with Their Bodies*, 26.

49. Ralph Harrington, "The Railway Accident," in *Traumatic Pasts: History, Psychiatry and Trauma in the Modern Age, 1870–1930*, ed. Mark S. Micale and Paul Lerner (New York: Cambridge University Press, 2001), 31–56, 34.

50. Paul Lerner and Mark S. Micale, "Trauma, Psychiatry, and History: A Conceptual and Historiographical Introduction," in ibid., 1–20, 9.

51. Harrington, "Railway Accident," in ibid., 45.

52. Quoted in Michael R. Trimble, *Post-Traumatic Neurosis: From Railway Spine to the Whiplash* (New York: John Wiley, 1981), 12.

53. Hacking, *Rewriting the Soul*, 186.

54. Trimble, *Post-Traumatic Neuroses*, 9.

55. Trimble, *Post-Traumatic Neuroses*, 3.

56. Quoted in Harrington, "Railway Accident," 45.

57. Trimble, *Post-Traumatic Neuroses*, 31.

58. Carl Weidner, "Traumatic Neurasthenia," *American Practitioner and News* 39 (1904): 410–20, 410–11.

59. Quoted in Trimble, *Post-Traumatic Neuroses*, 28.

60. Quoted in Trimble, *Post-Traumatic Neuroses*, 28.

61. Michael Roth, *Memory, Trauma, and History* (New York: Columbia University Press, 2012), 42.

62. Mark S. Micale, "Jean-Martin Charcot and *les neuroses traumatiques*," in Micale and Lerner, *Traumatic Pasts*, 115–139, 135 (see n49).

63. Lerner and Micale, "Trauma, Psychiatry, and History," in Micale and Lerner, *Traumatic Pasts*, 11. The term "nervous shock" became widely accepted, although the particular mechanisms through which it produced psychic symptoms were unknown. See also Hacking, *Rewriting the Soul*, 183.

64. Eric Caplan, "Trains and Trauma in the American Gilded Age," in Micale and Lerner, *Traumatic Pasts*, 57–80, 58.

65. Trimble, *Post-Traumatic Neuroses*, 30.

66. Trimble, *Post-Traumatic Neuroses*, 58.

67. Trimble, *Post-Traumatic Neuroses*, 64.

68. Caplan, "Trains and Trauma," 61.

69. Wolfgang Schaffner, "Event, Series, Trauma," in Micale and Lerner, *Traumatic Pasts*, 81–92, 83.

70. Harrington, "Railway Accident," 38–39.

71. Caplan, "Trains and Trauma," 68.

72. Greg A. Eghigian, "The German Welfare State as a Discourse of Trauma," in Micale and Lerner, *Traumatic Pasts*, 92–114, 106.

73. Eghigian, "German Welfare State," 106.

74. Paul Lerner, "From Traumatic Neurosis to Male Hysteria," in Micale and Lerner, *Traumatic Pasts*, 141.

75. Eghigian, "German Welfare State," 107, 108.

76. Eghigian, "German Welfare State," 110, and Lerner, "From Traumatic Neurosis to Male Hysteria," 150.

77. Henri F. Ellenberger, *The Discovery of the Unconscious: The History and Evolution of Dynamic Psychiatry* (New York: Basic Books, 1970), 46.

78. Roth, *Memory, Trauma, and History*, 43.

79. Allan Young, *The Harmony of Illusions: Inventing Post-Traumatic Stress Disorder* (Princeton, NJ: Princeton University Press, 1995), 29.

80. Ellenberger, *Discovery of the Unconscious*, 111.

81. "The past and where to keep it were being formed into a new problematic by doctors and philosophers ready to claim expertise about how much of a connection to the past was good for us," observes Michael Roth, in *Memory, Trauma, and History*, 21.

82. Micale, "Jean-Martin Charcot," 116.

83. Trimble, *Post-Traumatic Neuroses*, 45; Micale, "Jean-Martin Charcot," 120.

84. Young, *Harmony of Illusions*, 20.

85. The new medium of photography also provided public images of stereotypical hysterical symptoms that others could view and then copy and reinforce.

86. Paul R. McHugh, *Try to Remember: Psychiatry's Clash over Meaning, Memory, and Mind* (New York: Dana Press, 2008), 61.

87. Mark S. Micale, *Approaching Hysteria: Disease and Its Interpretations* (Princeton, NJ: Princeton University Press, 1995), 149.

88. Pierre Janet, *The Major Symptoms of Hysteria* (New York: Macmillan, 1920), 22.

89. Janet, *Major Symptoms of Hysteria*, 66–67.

90. Ellenberger, *Discovery of the Unconscious*, 344.

91. Janet, *Major Symptoms of Hysteria*, 291.

92. Janet, *Major Symptoms of Hysteria*, 141.

93. Ellenberger, *Discovery of the Unconscious*, 374.

94. Sigmund Freud, "On the Psychical Mechanism of Hysterical Phenomena," in Sigmund Freud, *Collected Papers*, ed. James Strachey, trans. Joan Riviere (1893; New York: Basic Books, 1959), 24–41, 25.

95. Micale, *Approaching Hysteria*, 66.

96. Sigmund Freud and Josef Breuer, *Three Studies on Hysteria*, trans. James and Alix Strachey (New York: Penguin, 1893/1974), 54.

97. Trimble, *Post-Traumatic Neuroses*, 49; Micale, *Approaching Hysteria*, 28.

98. Freud and Breuer, *Three Studies*, 58.

99. Sigmund Freud, "Some Points in a Comparative Study of Organic and Hysterical Paralysis," in Freud, *Collected Papers*, 42–58 (see n94); see also Micale, *Approaching Hysteria*, 182.

100. Sigmund Freud, "On the History of the Psycho-Analytic Movement," in Freud, *Collected Papers*, 287–359, 297 (see n94). Freud's formulations owed far more to Janet than he admitted. Janet derided Freud's position as derivative of his own, and they became bitter rivals (Ellenberger, *Discovery of the Unconscious*, 344). One difference between the two processes, however, is that dissociated memories remain in relatively pure form within the subconscious. In contrast, repressed memories are multilayered: "We have found out that no hysterical symptom can originate in one real experience alone, but that in every instance the memory roused by association co-operates with earlier experiences in causing the symptom." Freud, "The Aetiology of Hysteria," in Freud, *Collected Papers*, 190. Each discovery of a repressed trauma was not final but led to the exploration of even deeper layers of memory. Ultimately, however, patient recollections actually reproduced the original occurrence: "I was able to trace back, with certainty, a hysteria . . . to a seduction, which occurred for the first time at 11 months and [I could] hear again the words that were exchanged between two adults at that time! It is as though it comes from a photograph," Freud proclaimed in an 1897 letter to his friend Wilhelm Fliess. Quoted in Mikkel Borch-Jacobsen, "Self-Seduced," in *Unauthorized Freud*, ed. Frederick Crews (New York: Penguin, 1998), 43–53, 50.

101. Freud and Breuer, *Three Studies*, 60.

102. Freud and Breuer, *Three Studies*, 60; emphasis in original.

103. Freud and Breuer, *Three Studies*, 328; emphasis in original.

104. Sigmund Freud, "Heredity and the Aetiology of the Neuroses," in Freud, *Collected Papers*, 149; emphasis in original.

105. Freud, "Aetiology of Hysteria," in Freud, *Collected Papers*, 193; emphasis in original.

106. Sigmund Freud, "Further Remarks on the Defence Neuro-Psychoses," in Freud, *Collected Papers*, 156; emphasis in original.

107. John Kerr, *A Most Dangerous Method: The Story of Jung, Freud, and Sabina Spielrein* (New York: Vintage, 1993), 92.

108. George Makari, *Revolution in Mind: The Creation of Psychoanalysis* (New York: Harper, 2008), 88.

109. The well-known case of Sabina Spielrein, who went on to become a psychoanalyst as well as Carl Jung's lover, provides a good illustration of this phenomenon. She became sexually excited as a young child when she fantasized that her father was beating her. Kerr, *Most Dangerous Method*, 69, 120.

110. Freud, "Heredity," in Freud, *Collected Papers*, 151; emphasis in original.

111. Kerr, *Most Dangerous Method*, 78.

112. Sigmund Freud, "Further Remarks on the Defence Neuro-Psychoses," in Freud, *Collected Papers*, 157.

113. Sigmund Freud to Wilhelm Fliess, December 6, 1896, extract from the Fliess Papers, Letter 52, in *The Standard Edition of the Complete Psychological Works of Sigmund Freud*, ed. and trans. James Strachey (London: Hogarth Press, 1948), 1:233.

114. Sigmund Freud, "My Views on the Part Played by Sexuality in the Aetiology of the Neuroses," in Freud, *Collected Papers*, 276.

115. Sigmund Freud, *Introductory Lectures on Psycho-analysis (part III)*, in *Standard Edition of the Complete Psychological Works of Sigmund Freud* (1916–17; London: Liveright, 1989), 16:368.

116. Sigmund Freud, *The Interpretation of Dreams* (New York: Avon, 1965), 291.

117. Makari, *Revolution in Mind*, 98.

118. Freud and Breuer, *Three Studies*, 53.

119. Freud and Breuer, *Three Studies*, 74.

120. Freud and Breuer, *Three Studies*, 102. Breuer and Freud's stated belief that Anna O.'s symptoms disappeared was false. In fact, she was committed to a psychiatric hospital, and her problems persisted for a number of subsequent years.

121. Freud and Breuer, *Three Studies*, 299.

122. Freud and Breuer, "Psychical Mechanism," in Freud, *Collected Papers*, 28.

123. Freud, "Aetiology of Hysteria," 188.

124. Peter Gay, *Freud: A Life for Our Time* (New York: W. W. Norton, 1988), 50.

125. E.g., Mikkel Borch-Jacobsen, *Making Minds and Madness: From Hysteria to Depression* (New York: Cambridge University Press, 2009); Frank Cioffi, *Freud and the Question of Pseudoscience* (Chicago: Open Court, 1998); Frederick Crews, *Freud and the Making of an Illusion* (New York: Metropolitan Books, 2017); Allen Esterson, *Seductive Mirage: An Exploration of the Works of Sigmund Freud* (Chicago: Open Court, 1993); Richard J. McNally, *Remembering Trauma* (Cambridge, MA: Harvard University Press, 2003).

126. Sigmund Freud, "Fragment of an Analysis of a Case of Hysteria

('Dora')," in *The Freud Reader*, ed. Peter Gay (New York: W. W. Norton, 1989), 172–239, 203.

127. Gay, *Freud Reader*, 72.

128: Elizabeth Roudinesco, *Freud in His Time and Ours* (Cambridge, MA: Harvard University Press, 2016), 72.

129. Frederick Crews, "Introduction," in Crews, *Unauthorized Freud*, xvii–xxxi, xxviii.

130. Borch-Jacobsen, "Self-Seduced," in ibid., 46.

131. Freud, "Heredity and Aetiology," in Freud, *Collected Papers*, 150.

132. Richard Ofshe and Ethan Watters, *Making Monsters* (Berkeley: University of California Press, 1994), 291.

Chapter 3. The Psychic Wounds of Combat

1. Nathan G. Hale, *The Rise and Crisis of Psychoanalysis in the United States* (New York: Oxford University Press, 1995), 15. Two-thirds of the American soldiers who were evacuated for psychiatric reasons never returned to combat. John M. Kinder, *Paying with Their Bodies: American War and the Problem of the Disabled Veteran* (Chicago: University of Chicago Press, 2015), 67. Over the course of war, about 40 percent of discharges of British soldiers were related to psychiatric issues. Andrew Scull, *Madness in Civilization* (Princeton, NJ: Princeton University Press, 2015), 337.

2. Chris Feudtner, "'Minds the Dead Have Ravished': Shell Shock, History, and the Ecology of Disease-Systems," *History of Science* 31 (1993): 377–420.

3. The focus on shell shock was most common among the British; French psychiatrists were more likely to consider the condition a form of hysteria. Ben Shephard, *A War of Nerves: Soldiers and Psychiatrists in the Twentieth Century* (Cambridge, MA: Harvard University Press, 2000), 97.

4. Franklin D. Jones, "Military Psychiatry since World War II," in *American Psychiatry after World War II: 1944–1994*, ed. Roy W. Menninger and John C. Nemiah (Washington, DC: American Psychiatric Press, 2000), 3–36, 4.

5. Shephard, *War of Nerves*, 174. Subsequent studies of World War I case registers show how little resemblance existed between the symptoms of shell-shocked soldiers and current features of PTSD, which are marked by intrusive reexperiencing of the trauma, emotional blunting, and hyperarousal. Lars Weisaeth, "The History of Psychic Trauma," in *Handbook of PTSD*, ed. Matthew J. Friedman, Terence M. Keane, and Patricia A. Resick (New York: Guilford Press, 2014), 38–59, 47.

6. Quoted in Jones, "Military Psychiatry," in Menninger and Nemiah, *American Psychiatry*, 3.

7. Shephard, *War of Nerves*, 140.

8. Quoted in Shephard, *War of Nerves*, 31.

9. Quoted in Jerry Lembcke, *The Spitting Image: Myth, Memory, and the Legacy of Vietnam* (New York: New York University Press, 1998), 69.

10. Edgar Jones and Simon Wessely, *Shell Shock to PTSD: Military Psychiatry from 1900 to the Gulf War* (New York: Psychology Press, 2005), 21.

11. There were considerable differences in the symptomatic presentations of shell shock across different national armies. For example, German soldiers were far more likely to display traditional symptoms of hysteria than the French. Scull, *Madness in Civilization*, 297.

12. Kinder, *Paying with Their Bodies*, 58–59.

13. Jones and Wessely, *Shell Shock to PTSD*, 52.

14. Peter Leese, "'Why Are They Not Cured?': British Shellshock Treatment during the Great War," in *Traumatic Pasts: History, Psychiatry, and Trauma in the Modern Age, 1870–1930*, ed. Mark S. Micale and Paul Lerner (New York: Cambridge University Press, 2001), 205–221, 217.

15. Fischer-Homberger, quoted in Jose Brunner, "Will, Desire, and Experience," *Transcultural Psychiatry* 37 (2000): 295–320, 304.

16. Brunner, "Will, Desire, and Experience."

17. Quoted in Shephard, *War of Nerves*, 111.

18. Sándor Ferenczi, Karl Abraham, Ernst Simmel, and Ernest Jones, *Psycho-analysis and the War Neuroses* (London: International Psycho-Analytical Press, 1919).

19. Dixon Wecter, *When Johnny Comes Marching Home* (Cambridge, MA: Houghton Mifflin, 1944), 390–391.

20. See especially Allan Young, *The Harmony of Illusions: Inventing Post-Traumatic Stress Disorder* (Princeton, NJ: Princeton University Press, 1995), 43–61.

21. Freud objected to the portrayal of shell-shocked soldiers as malingerers and did not regard simulation as a common problem. Henri F. Ellenberger, *The Discovery of the Unconscious: The History and Evolution of Dynamic Psychiatry* (New York: Basic Books, 1970), 837–838.

22. "Introduction to Psycho-analysis and the War Neurosis," in *The Standard Edition of the Complete Psychological Works of Sigmund Freud*, ed. and trans. James Strachey (London: Hogarth Press, 1955), 17:210.

23. Sigmund Freud, *Beyond the Pleasure Principle*, trans. James Strachey (New York: W. W. Norton, 1989), 33.

24. John P. Wilson, "The Historical Evolution of PTSD Diagnostic Criteria: From Freud to DSM-IV," *Journal of Traumatic Stress* 7 (1994): 681–698.

25. Sigmund Freud, *Introductory Lectures on Psychoanalysis*, trans. James Strachey (1916; New York: W. W. Norton, 1989), 274–275.

26. American Psychiatric Association, *Diagnostic and Statistical Manual of Mental Disorders*, 3rd ed. (Washington, DC: American Psychiatric Association, 1980), 238.

27. Sigmund Freud, *New Introductory Lectures on Psychoanalysis*, trans. James Strachey (1933; New York: W. W. Norton, 1965), 28.

28. Freud, *Beyond the Pleasure Principle*, 11.

29. George Makari, *Revolution in Mind: The Creation of Psychoanalysis* (New York: Harper, 2008), 317.

30. Freud, *Introductory Lectures on Psychoanalysis*, 275.

31. Shephard, *War of Nerves*, 71. Newspapers, too, depicted shell-shocked soldiers as "deranged lunatics prone to violence and fits of hysteria." Kinder, *Paying with Their Bodies*, 101.

32. Young, *Harmony of Illusions*, 68–72.

33. Hale, *Rise and Crisis*, 21. The French, however, focused on uncovering supposed malingerers and quickly getting them back to the battlefield. Shephard, *War of Nerves*, 102.

34. Elaine Showalter, *The Female Malady: Women, Madness, and English Culture, 1830–1980* (New York: Pantheon, 1985), 189.

35. Shephard, *War of Nerves*.

36. Shephard, *War of Nerves*, 47.

37. Jones and Wessely, *Shell Shock to PTSD*, 21.

38. Shephard, *War of Nerves*, 59.

39. Quoted in Shephard, *War of Nerves*, 129.

40. Shephard, *War of Nerves*, 29.

41. Ian Kershaw, *To Hell and Back: Europe, 1914–1949* (New York: Viking, 2015), 98.

42. Jay Winter, "Shell-shock and the Cultural History of the Great War," *Journal of Contemporary History* 35 (2000): 7–11.

43. Quoted in Shephard, *War of Nerves*, 89.

44. Robert Graves, *Goodbye to All That* (New York: Vintage, 1998), 287, 289.

45. Virginia Woolf, *Mrs. Dalloway* (1925; London: Chancellor Press, 1994), 216.

46. Willard W. Waller, *The Veteran Comes Back* (1944; San Francisco: Forgotten Books, 2006), 109.

47. Quoted in Shephard, *War of Nerves*, 144.

48. Quoted in Michael R. Trimble, *Post-Traumatic Neurosis: From Railway Spine to the Whiplash* (New York: John Wiley, 1981), 98.

49. Abram Kardiner, *Traumatic Neuroses of War* (New York: Harper & Brothers, 1941).

50. Kardiner, *Traumatic Neuroses*, 91–93.

51. Kardiner, *Traumatic Neuroses*, 123–124.

52. Kardiner, *Traumatic Neuroses*, 88.

53. Kardiner, *Traumatic Neuroses*, 137.

54. Kardiner, *Traumatic Neuroses*, 5.

55. Kardiner, *Traumatic Neuroses*, 218.

56. Kardiner, *Traumatic Neuroses*, 232.

57. Kardiner, *Traumatic Neuroses*, 235.

58. Kardiner, *Traumatic Neuroses*, 236.

59. Kardiner, *Traumatic Neuroses*, 189.

60. Kardiner, *Traumatic Neuroses*, 190.

61. Jones and Wessely, *Shell Shock to PTSD*, 144.

62. Quoted in Jones and Wessely, *Shell Shock to PTSD*, 54, 151. Edgar Jones, Ian Palmer, and Simon Wessely, "War Pensions (1900–1945): Changing Models of Psychological Understanding," *British Journal of Psychiatry* 180 (2002): 374–379, 376.

63. Shephard, *War of Nerves*, 167.

64. Weisaeth, "History of Psychic Trauma," in Friedman, Keane, and Resick, *Handbook of PTSD*, 45 (see n5).

65. Quoted in Jones and Wessely, *Shell Shock to PTSD*, 156.

66. Scull, *Madness in Civilization*, 336.

67. Kinder, *Paying with Their Bodies*, 86.

68. Shephard, *War of Nerves*, 153.

69. Caroline Cox, "Invisible Wounds: The American Legion, Shell-Shocked Veterans, and American Society, 1919–1924," in Micale and Lerner, *Traumatic Pasts*, 280–305, 291 (see n14).

70. Kinder, *Paying with Their Bodies*, 184.

71. Kinder, *Paying with Their Bodies*, 147.

72. Kinder, *Paying with Their Bodies*, 5.

73. Wecter, *When Johnny Comes Marching Home*, 403.

74. Kinder, *Paying with Their Bodies*, 176.

75. Erin Finley, *Fields of Combat: Understanding PTSD among Veterans of Iraq and Afghanistan* (Ithaca, NY: IRL Press), 92.

76. Waller, *Veteran Comes Back*, 168, 267.

77. Wecter, *When Johnny Comes Marching Home*, 404.

78. Kinder, *Paying with Their Bodies*, 164, 197.

79. Shephard, *War of Nerves*, 165.

80. Shephard, *War of Nerves*, 151; Kinder, *Paying with Their Bodies*, 3–4.

81. Shephard, *War of Nerves*, 169–171; Jones and Wessely, *Shell Shock to PTSD*, 70.

82. Gerald N. Grob, *From Asylum to Community: Mental Health Policy in Modern America* (Princeton, NJ: Princeton University Press, 1991), 17.

83. Jones and Wessely, *Shell Shock to PTSD*, 104.

84. Ellen Herman, *The Romance of American Psychology* (Berkeley: University of California Press, 1995), 87.

85. Jones, "Military Psychiatry," 7.

86. John Aita, "Efficacy of Brief Clinical Interview Method in Predict-

ing Adjustment: Five-year Follow-up Study of 304 Army Inductees," *Archives of Neurology and Psychiatry* 61 (1949): 170–178.

87. Grob, *Asylum to Community*, 14.

88. Shephard, *War of Nerves*.

89. Shephard, *War of Nerves*, 201.

90. Grob, *Asylum to Community*, 13; Herman, *Romance of American Psychology*, 89.

91. Grob, *Asylum to Community*, 13.

92. Shephard, *War of Nerves*, 327.

93. Hale, *Rise and Crisis*, 204.

94. Shephard, *War of Nerves*, 235.

95. Herbert Spiegel, "Silver Linings in the Clouds of War: A Five-Decade Retrospective," in *American Psychiatry after World War II: 1944–1994*, ed. Roy W. Menninger and John C. Nemiah (Washington, DC: American Psychiatric Association, 2000), 52–72, 58.

96. Roy R. Grinker and John P. Spiegel, *Men under Stress* (Philadelphia: Blakeston, 1945).

97. The varying conditions of combat during the two wars could also have influenced symptom presentations: the alternation of passive waiting in trenches with horrifying artillery barrages or charges into enemy lines could be more congruent with hysterical symptoms, while the less confined situations of most soldiers in the latter war could be more conducive to depressive and anxious symptoms.

98. Jones, "Military Psychiatry," 8.

99. Grob, *Asylum to Community*.

100. Rates of psychiatric breakdowns were closely correlated with the total number of physically wounded soldiers, indicating that the conditions of battle themselves rather than predispositions were associated with higher amounts of combat neuroses. Jones and Wessely, *Shell Shock to PTSD*, 118.

101. Roy R. Grinker and John P. Spiegel, *War Neuroses in North Africa* (New York: Air Surgeon, Army Air Forces, 1943), 115.

102. Gilbert Beebe and John Apple, "Psychological Breakdown in Relation to Stress and Other Factors," in *Variation in Psychological Tolerance to Ground Combat in World War II* (Washington, DC: National Academy of Science, 1958), 88–131.

103. Roy Swank and Walter Marchand, "Combat Neuroses: Development of Combat Exhaustion," *Archives of Neurology and Psychiatry* 55 (1946): 236–247, 243, 244.

104. John Keegan, *The Face of Battle* (New York: Penguin, 1976), 329.

105. Shephard, *War of Nerves*, 326.

106. Quoted in Wecter, *When Johnny Comes Marching Home*, 546.

107. Shephard, *War of Nerves*, 215; Hale, *Rise and Crisis*, 191.

108. Winter, "Shell-shock," 65.

109. Shephard, *War of Nerves*, 224–225.

110. Shephard, *War of Nerves*, 216, 226.

111. Quoted in Grob, *Asylum to Community*, 16.

112. Wecter, *When Johnny Comes Marching Home*, 547.

113. Grob, *Asylum to Community*, 16; Shephard, *War of Nerves*, 255.

114. Jones and Wessely, *Shell Shock to PTSD*, 88.

115. Jones and Wessely, *Shell Shock to PTSD*, 79, 84.

116. Quoted in Shephard, *War of Nerves*, 202.

117. Winter, "Shell-shock," 107.

118. Waller, *Veteran Comes Back*, 166.

119. Waller, *Veteran Comes Back*, 110.

120. Waller, *Veteran Comes Back*, 180. Dixon Wecter's 1944 book, *When Johnny Comes Marching Home*, similarly highlights veterans' difficulties with jobs, income, and social relationships and gives short shrift to lingering psychological problems.

121. Waller, *Veteran Comes Back*, 59.

122. Waller, *Veteran Comes Back*, 173.

123. Waller, *Veteran Comes Back*, 13.

124. Scull, *Madness in Civilization*, 338; Shephard, *War of Nerves*, 330.

125. Shephard, *War of Nerves*, 330. In Britain, 10 percent of all pensions were awarded for psychological disorders after World War II, well above the 6 percent that were given for this reason after World War I. Jones and Wessely, *Shell Shock to PTSD*, 160.

126. Almost all prisoners of war, half of whom displayed psychiatric symptoms after release, were soon involved in successful careers and stable family lives. Eric T. Dean Jr., *Shook over Hell: Post-Traumatic Stress, Vietnam, and the Civil War* (Cambridge, MA: Harvard University Press, 1991), 199.

127. Hans Pols, "The Repression of War Trauma in American Psychiatry after WWII," in *Medicine and Modern Warfare*, ed. Roger Cooter, Mark Harrison, and Steve Sturdy (Leiden: Clio Medica, 1999), 251–276, 270.

128. Kinder, *Paying with Their Bodies*, 267.

129. Sloan Wilson, *The Man in the Gray Flannel Suit* (1955; New York: Da Capo Press, 2002), 86, 97, 98, 126.

130. See https://www.wwiimemorial.com/dedication/speeches/Dedication-Brokaw.htm, retrieved September 17, 2017.

Chapter 4. Diagnosing PTSD

1. William C. Menninger, "Psychiatric Experience in the War, 1941–1956," *American Journal of Psychiatry* 103 (1947): 577–586, 580.

2. E.g., Michael E. Staub, *Madness Is Civilization: When the Diagnosis Was Social: 1948–1980* (Chicago: University of Chicago Press, 2011).

3. Gerald N. Grob, *From Asylum to Community* (Princeton, NJ: Princeton University Press, 1991), 18.

4. Robert H. Felix and R. V. Bowers, "Mental Hygiene and Socio-Environmental Factors," *Milbank Memorial Fund Quarterly* 26 (1948): 125–147, 125.

5. American Psychiatric Association, *The Statistical Manual for the Use of Hospitals for Mental Diseases* (Utica, NY: State Hospitals Press, 1942), 29.

6. William C. Menninger, "Lessons from Military Psychiatry for Civilian Psychiatry," *Mental Hygiene* 40 (1946): 581.

7. Nolan Lewis and Bernice Engle, *Wartime Psychiatry* (Oxford: Oxford University Press, 1954).

8. William C. Menninger, "War Department Bulletin, *Medical 203*" (Washington, DC: Army Service Forces, 1943).

9. Nathan G. Hale, *The Rise and Crisis of Psychoanalysis in the United States* (New York: Oxford University Press, 1995), 200.

10. Grob, *Asylum to Community*, 97.

11. American Psychiatric Association, *Diagnostic and Statistical Manual of Mental Disorders* (Washington, DC: American Psychiatric Association, 1952), 16, 20.

12. *Diagnostic and Statistical Manual*, vi.

13. *Diagnostic and Statistical Manual*, vii.

14. *Diagnostic and Statistical Manual*, 40.

15. *Diagnostic and Statistical Manual*, 40.

16. American Psychiatric Association, *Diagnostic and Statistical Manual of Mental Disorders*, 2nd ed. (Washington, DC: American Psychiatric Association, 1968), 48.

17. *DSM-II*, 49.

18. Paul Starr, *The Discarded Army: Veterans after Vietnam* (New York: Charterhouse, 1973), 24.

19. Edgar Jones and Simon Wessely, *Shell Shock to PTSD: Military Psychiatry from 1900 to the Gulf War* (New York: Psychology Press, 2005), 128.

20. Ben Shephard, *A War of Nerves: Soldiers and Psychiatrists in the Twentieth Century* (Cambridge, MA: Harvard University Press, 2000), 340.

21. Peter G. Bourne, "Military Psychiatry and the Viet Nam Experience," *American Journal of Psychiatry* 127 (1970): 481–488, 487.

22. John E. Helzer, Lee N. Robins, and Darlene H. Davis, "Depressive Disorders in Vietnam Returnees," *Journal of Nervous and Mental Disorders* 168 (1976): 177–185.

23. J. F. Borus, "Incidence of Maladjustment in Vietnam Returnees," *Archives of General Psychiatry* 30 (1974): 554–557.

24. John E. Helzer, Lee N. Robins, and Darlene H. Davis, "Antecedents of Narcotic Use and Addiction: A Study of 898 Vietnam Veterans," *Drug and Alcohol Dependence* 1 (1976): 183–193.

25. Starr, *Discarded Army*, 1973.

26. Eric T. Dean Jr., *Shook over Hell: Post-Traumatic Stress, Vietnam, and the Civil War* (Cambridge, MA: Harvard University Press, 1991), 18.

27. Dean, *Shook over Hell*, 12–13, 186. Similarly, by 1978 veterans made up half of the federal government workforce, double the national average for all jobs.

28. Dean, *Shook over Hell*, 190.

29. Jerry Lembcke, *PTSD: Diagnosis and Identity in Post-empire America* (New York: Lexington, 2013), 107. For example, the popular film *Airplane*, released in 1980, the same year as the *DSM-III*, portrays a traumatized veteran who flashes back to his experiences in Vietnam.

30. Quoted in Dean, *Shook over Hell*, 24. Such flashback-like phenomena were rarely recorded among veterans of previous wars. Jones and Wessely's study of 567 World War I veterans found only 3 cases in which flashbacks were described; their study of 367 World War II pensioners uncovered just 5 who reported flashbacks (*Shell Shock to PTSD*, 174).

31. Dean, *Shook over Hell*, 183.

32. Jonathan Shay, *Achilles in Vietnam: Combat Trauma and the Undoing of Character* (New York: Scribner, 1994), 7.

33. Nancy Andreasen, "Posttraumatic Stress Disorder: Psychology, Biology, and the Manichean Warfare between False Dichotomies," *American Journal of Psychiatry* 152 (1995): 964.

34. Dean, *Shook over Hell*, 9.

35. Cited in Jerry Lembcke, *The Spitting Image: Myth, Memory, and the Legacy of Vietnam* (New York: New York University Press, 1998), 47.

36. Lembcke, *PTSD*, 116.

37. Dean, *Shook over Hell*, 21.

38. Wilbur J. Scott, "PTSD in *DSM-III*: A Case in the Politics of Diagnosis and Disease," *Social Problems* 37 (1990): 294–310.

39. Wilbur J. Scott, *Vietnam Veterans since the War* (Norman: University of Oklahoma Press, 2004), 15. One VA psychologist observed "an almost neurotic need to regard the Vietnam veteran as being traumatized by the war." Robert Fleming, "Post Vietnam Syndrome: Neurosis or Sociosis?," *Psychiatry* 48 (1985): 122–139, 123.

40. Bruno Bettelheim, "Individual and Mass Behavior in Extreme Situations," *Journal of Abnormal and Social Psychology* 38 (1943): 417–452.

41. Bettelheim, "Behavior in Extreme Situations," in ibid.

42. Shephard, *A War of Nerves*, 360–361.

43. William G. Niederland, *The Problems of the Survivor: Part I, Journal of the Hillside Hospital* 10 (1961): 233–247.

44. Many VA psychiatrists, in turn, belittled these groups, which one characterized as creating a "ghetto-like environment [that] isolates the mal-

adjusted veteran from society" (Fleming, "Post Vietnam Syndrome," 138). In their view, rap groups "abet rather than alleviate" existing problems of adjustment and reinforce veterans' alienation.

45. David Morris, *The Evil Hours: A Biography of Post-Traumatic Stress Disorder* (Boston: Houghton Mifflin Harcourt, 2015), 144.

46. Robert J. Lifton, *Home from the War* (New York: Simon & Schuster, 1973), 219.

47. Lifton, *Home from the War*, 94.

48. Lifton, *Home from the War*, 238.

49. Chaim Shatan, "Post-Vietnam Syndrome," *New York Times*, May 6, 1972.

50. Quoted in B. G. Burkett and Glenna Whitley, *Stolen Valor: How the Vietnam Generation Was Robbed of Its Heroes and Its History* (Dallas: Verity Press, 1998), 142.

51. Robert Jay Lifton, "From Hiroshima to the Nazi Doctors," in *International Handbook of Traumatic Stress Syndromes*, ed. John P. Wilson and Beverley Raphael (New York: Plenum Press, 1993), 11–23, 18.

52. Lifton, "From Hiroshima to the Nazi Doctors," in ibid., 11, 16.

53. Starr, *Discarded Army*, 35.

54. Quoted in Scott, "PTSD in *DSM-III*," 28.

55. Sarah Haley, "When the Patient Reports Atrocities: Specific Treatment Considerations of the Vietnam Veteran," *Archives of General Psychiatry* 30 (1974): 191–196, 191.

56. Gerald Nicosia, *Home to War: A History of the Vietnam Veterans' Movement* (New York: Three Rivers Press, 2001), 171.

57. Burkett and Whitley, *Stolen Valor*, 142.

58. Quoted in Jones and Wessely, *Shell Shock to PTSD*, 135.

59. Richard B. Fuller, "War Veterans' Post-traumatic Stress Disorder and the U.S. Congress," in *Post-Traumatic Stress Disorder and the War Veteran Patient*, ed. W. E. Kelly (New York: Brunner/Mazel, 1985), 3–11.

60. Jones and Wessely, *Shell Shock to PTSD*, 131.

61. Shephard, *War of Nerves*, 360.

62. Charles E. Rosenberg, *Our Present Complaint: American Medicine, Then and Now* (Baltimore: Johns Hopkins University Press, 2007), 13.

63. Allan V. Horwitz, *Creating Mental Illness* (Chicago: University of Chicago Press, 2002).

64. Scott, *Vietnam Veterans*, 64; Lifton, "From Hiroshima to the Nazi Doctors," 17.

65. Helzer, Robins, and Davis, "Antecedents"; Helzer, Robins, and Davis, "Depressive Disorders."

66. Michael R. Hryvniak and Richard Rosse, "Concurrent Psychiatric

Illness in Inpatients with Post-Traumatic Stress Disorder," *Military Medicine* 154 (1989): 399–401.

67. John P. Wilson, "The Historical Evolution of PTSD Diagnostic Criteria: From Freud to DSM-IV," *Journal of Traumatic Stress* 7 (1994): 681–698.

68. Chaim F. Shatan, "Have You Hugged a Vietnam Veteran Today? The Basic Wound of Catastrophic Stress," in Kelly, *Post-Traumatic Stress Disorder*, 12–28, 21 (see n59).

69. Abram Kardiner, *Traumatic Neuroses of War* (New York: Harper & Brothers, 1941), 237.

70. E.g., N. C. Andreasen and A. S. Norris, "Long-term Adjustment and Adaptation Mechanisms in Severely Burned Adults," *Journal of Nervous and Mental Disorders* 154 (1972): 352–362; N. C. Andreasen, A. S. Norris, and C. E. Hartford, "Incidence of Long-term Psychiatric Complications in Severely Burned Adults," *Annals of Surgery* 174 (1971): 785–795.

71. Scott, "PTSD in *DSM-III*."

72. Allan Young, *The Harmony of Illusions: Inventing Post-Traumatic Stress Disorder* (Princeton, NJ: Princeton University Press, 1995); Herb Kutchins and Stuart A. Kirk, *Making Us Crazy: DSM: The Psychiatric Bible and the Creation of Mental Disorders* (New York: Free Press, 1997), 107–123.

73. Scott, "PTSD in *DSM-III*," 308.

74. American Psychiatric Association, *Diagnostic and Statistical Manual of Mental Disorders*, 3rd ed. (Washington, DC: American Psychiatric Association, 1980), 238.

75. *DSM-III*, 237.

76. *DSM-III*, 236.

77. Hannah S. Decker, *The Making of DSM-III: A Diagnostic Manual's Conquest of American Psychiatry* (Oxford: Oxford University Press, 2013), xv.

78. *DSM-III*, 238.

79. *DSM-III*, 237.

80. Lifton noted that "Kardiner's thinking closely approximates our own." "From Hiroshima to the Nazi Doctors," 15.

81. Shephard, *War of Nerves*, 157.

82. Sigmund Freud, *Beyond the Pleasure Principle*, trans. James Strachey (New York: W. W. Norton, 1989), 25.

83. Kardiner, *Traumatic Neuroses*, 79.

84. Kardiner, *Traumatic Neuroses*, 3.

85. Kardiner, *Traumatic Neuroses*, 176.

86. Nicosia, *Home to War*, 208. Others contend that the most notable quality of the symptom criteria—the dramatic reexperiencing of past traumatic events in the present—was actually drawn from media presentations.

Sociologist Jerry Lembcke asserts that "filmmakers thus virtually created the definition of a flashback as a trauma-induced, mental phenomenon." Lembcke, *PTSD*, 107.

87. Decker, *Making of DSM-III*, 117. In her 2001 book, *Brave New Brain*, Andreasen claims that "working with representatives of the Vietnam veterans, I developed the set of diagnostic criteria that defined what came to be known as PTSD" (305–306). She emphasizes how her burn patients "would frequently relive the catastrophe, suffer recurrent nightmares, have an exaggerated startle response, or retreat from their experience and show 'psychic numbing.'" Her published work, however, focuses on the depression, anxiety, phobias, and delirium that her burn victims suffered.

88. *DSM-III*, 238; Freud, *Beyond the Pleasure Principle*.

89. Kardiner, *Traumatic Neuroses*, 248.

90. Mardi J. Horowitz, *Image Formation and Cognition* (New York: Appleton-Century-Crofts, 1970).

91. Mardi J. Horowitz and G. F. Solomon, "A Prediction of Stress Response Syndromes in Vietnam Veterans," *Journal of Social Issues* 31 (1975): 67–80, 68.

92. Mardi J. Horowitz, *Stress Response Syndromes* (New York: Jason Aronson, 1976), 58.

93. Freud, quoted in Young, *Harmony of Illusions*, 78.

94. Kardiner, *Traumatic Neuroses*, 209, 210.

95. Horowitz, *Stress Response Syndromes*, 38.

96. Horowitz and Solomon, "Prediction of Stress Response Syndromes," 69.

97. John C. O'Donnell, "Military Service and Mental Health in Later Life," *Military Medicine* 165 (2000): 219–223.

98. Paula P. Schnurr, Avron Spiro, Melanie J. Vielhauer, Marianne N. Findler, and Jessica L. Hamblen, "Trauma in the Lives of Older Men: Findings from the Normative Aging Study," *Journal of Clinical Geropsychology* 8 (2002): 175–187.

99. Kimberly A. Lee, George E. Vaillant, William C. Torrey, and Glen H. Elder, "A 50-year Prospective Study of the Psychological Sequelae of World War II Combat," *American Journal of Psychiatry* 152 (1995): 516–522.

100. Jones and Wessely, *Shell Shock to PTSD*, 181.

101. Jones and Wessely, *Shell Shock to PTSD*, 182, 184.

102. Centers for Disease Control Vietnam Experience Study, "Health Status of Vietnam Veterans: I. Psychosocial Characteristics," *Journal of the American Medical Association* 259 (1988): 2701–2707, 2705.

103. John E. Helzer, Lee N. Robins, and Larry McEvoy, "Post-Traumatic Stress Disorder in the General Population," *New England Journal of Medicine* 317 (1987): 1630–1634.

104. Jonathan R. Davidson, Dana Hughes, Dan G. Blazer, and Linda K. George, "Post-traumatic Stress Disorder in the Community," *Psychological Medicine* 21 (1991): 713–721.

105. Allan Young and Naomi Breslau, "Troublesome Memories: Reflections on the Future," *Journal of Anxiety Disorders* 21 (2007): 230–232.

106. Paul R. McHugh, *Try to Remember: Psychiatry's Clash over Meaning, Memory, and Mind* (New York: Dana Press, 2008).

107. Lembcke, *Spitting Image*, 58.

Chapter 5. The Return of the Repressed

1. E.g., Catherine MacKinnon, *Feminism Unmodified: Discourses on Life and Law* (Cambridge, MA: Harvard University Press, 1988); Andrea Dworkin, *Intercourse* (New York: Basic Books, 1987); Gloria Steinem, *Outrageous Acts and Everyday Rebellions* (New York: Henry Holt, 1983).

2. Quoted in Richard Ofshe and Ethan Watters, *Making Monsters: False Memories, Psychotherapy, and Sexual Hysteria* (Berkeley: University of California Press, 1994), 10. Feminist issues were paradoxically joined to those of the advocates of conservative values who gained prominence during the presidency of Ronald Reagan (1981–89). This group was alarmed by the growing numbers of women entering the work force, rising rates of divorce, expanding proportions of children placed in day care, and the consequent weakening of nuclear families. The unlikely result was a convergence of the concerns of radical feminists and those of Christian fundamentalists, which shaped the development of the recovered memory movement that emerged in the 1980s. Joan Acocella, *Creating Hysteria: Women and Multiple Personality Disorder* (San Francisco: Jossey-Bass, 1999).

3. Diana E. Russell, *The Secret Trauma: Incest in the Lives of Girls and Women*, rev. ed. (New York: Basic Books, 1999), 30.

4. Judith L. Herman, *Father-Daughter Incest* (Cambridge, MA: Harvard University Press, 1981), 4. "Violence," Herman also claimed, "is a routine part of women's sexual and domestic lives." Judith Herman, *Trauma and Recovery: The Aftermath of Violence—From Domestic Abuse to Political Terror* (New York: Basic Books, 2015), 28.

5. Sue Blume, *Secret Survivors: Uncovering Incest and Its Aftereffects in Women* (New York: John Wiley & Sons, 1990); Renee Fredrickson, *Repressed Memories: A Journey to Recovery from Sexual Abuse* (Seattle: Parkside, 1992).

6. Frederick Crews, *The Memory Wars: Freud's Legacy in Dispute* (New York: New York Review of Books, 1995), 232.

7. Crews, *Memory Wars*, 159.

8. Herman, *Trauma and Recovery*, 122.

9. Fredrickson, *Repressed Memories*, 15.

10. Herman, *Trauma and Recovery*, 28.

11. Paul R. McHugh, *Try to Remember: Psychiatry's Clash over Meaning, Memory, and Mind* (New York: Dana Press, 2008), 177.

12. Bessel A. van der Kolk, *Psychological Trauma* (Washington, DC: American Psychiatric Press, 1987); Lenore Terr, *Unchained Memories: True Stories of Traumatic Memories, Lost and Found* (New York: Basic Books, 1994).

13. Ofshe and Watters, *Making Monsters*, 25–36.

14. Alison Winter, *Memory: Fragments of a Modern History* (Chicago: University of Chicago Press, 2012).

15. See Chap. 3. Although it loathed much of Freud's work, in many respects the RMM resurrected his initial theories about the causes of traumatic hysteria. For both, the most impactful traumas were ones that occurred in infancy or childhood. Likewise, their explanations of traumatic symptoms focused on repressed memories of sexual abuse. As well, each used hypnotic and other therapies to recover unconscious recollections of past traumas. Finally, both involved strong currents of suggestion to uncover these repressed memories of early abuse. Nonetheless, there are also differences between the RMM and Freud's early views of trauma-related illnesses. The RMM was almost uniquely American, as opposed to the European roots of Freud's infatuation with repressed memories. In addition, Freud's typically wealthy and Jewish clientele could hardly have differed more from the working- and middle-class, often evangelical, Christians who recovered traumatic memories during the 1980s. Finally—in contrast to Freud's first patients, who would have confronted an unfamiliar type of explanation for their symptoms—clients and clinicians associated with the RMM shared a therapeutic culture that was highly attuned to explanations associating distressing symptoms with early childhood victimization.

16. Quoted in Acocella, *Creating Hysteria*, 36.

17. Quoted in Dagmar Herzog, *Cold War Freud: Psychoanalysis in an Age of Catastrophes* (New York: Cambridge University Press, 2017), 218.

18. Sigmund Freud, "The Aetiology of Hysteria," in *The Freud Reader*, ed. Peter Gay (New York: W. W. Norton, 1989), 96–111, 103.

19. Quoted in John Kerr, *A Most Dangerous Method: The Story of Jung, Freud, and Sabina Spielrein* (New York: Vintage, 1993), 37–38.

20. Jeffrey Masson, *The Assault on Truth: Freud's Suppression of the Seduction Theory* (New York: Farrar, Straus & Giroux, 1984).

21. Herman, *Trauma and Recovery*, 13.

22. Herman, *Trauma and Recovery*, 14.

23. Herman, *Trauma and Recovery*; Onno van der Hart, Paul Brown, and Bessel A. van der Kolk, "Pierre Janet's Treatment of Post-Traumatic Stress," *Journal of Traumatic Stress* 2 (1989): 379–395.

24. Ian Hacking, "Memory Sciences, Memory Politics," in *Tense Past:*

Cultural Essays in Trauma and Memory, ed. Paul Antze and Michael Lambek (London: Routledge, 1996), 67–88, 76.

25. Pierre Janet, *The Major Symptoms of Hysteria* (New York: Macmillan, 1920), 66.

26. Mikkel Borch-Jacobsen, *Making Minds and Madness: From Hysteria to Depression* (New York: Cambridge University Press, 2009), 64.

27. Ian Hacking, *Rewriting the Soul: Multiple Personality and the Sciences of Memory* (Princeton, NJ: Princeton University Press, 1995), 46.

28. Hacking, *Rewriting the Soul*, 82.

29. Elaine Showalter, *Hystories: Hysterical Epidemics and Modern Media* (New York: Columbia University Press, 1997), 161.

30. Herman, *Trauma and Recovery*, 74, 87.

31. Showalter, *Hystories*; Acocella, *Creating Hysteria*.

32. Ellen Bass and Laura Davis, *The Courage to Heal: A Guide for Women Survivors of Sexual Abuse* (New York: William Morrow, 1988), 18.

33. Roger Luckhurst, *The Trauma Question* (New York: Routledge, 2008), 72.

34. Bass and Davis, *Courage to Heal*, 22.

35. Mikkel Borch-Jacobsen, "Anna O: The First Tall Tale," in *Unauthorized Freud: Doubters Confront a Legend*, ed. Frederick Crews (New York: Penguin, 1998), 10–21, 13.

36. Ofshe and Watters, *Making Monsters*, 145.

37. Herman, *Trauma and Recovery*, 1.

38. Michael Roth, *Memory, Trauma, and History* (New York: Columbia University Press, 2012), 96.

39. Bass and Davis, *Courage to Heal*, 135, 139.

40. Winter, *Memory*, 191.

41. Winter, *Memory*, 5.

42. Ofshe and Watters, *Making Monsters*, 177.

43. Herman, *Trauma and Recovery*, 240.

44. Herman, *Trauma and Recovery*, 7, 178.

45. American Psychiatric Association, *Diagnostic and Statistical Manual of Mental Disorders*, 3rd ed. (Washington, DC: American Psychiatric Association, 1980), 238.

46. Herman, *Trauma and Recovery*, 1.

47. Herman, *Trauma and Recovery*, 121.

48. Bessel A. van der Kolk and Mark S. Greenberg, "The Psychobiology of the Trauma Response," in *Psychological Trauma*, ed. Bessel van der Kolk (Washington, DC: American Psychiatric Press, 1987), 63–88.

49. American Psychiatric Association, *Diagnostic and Statistical Manual of Mental Disorders*, 3rd ed., rev. (Washington, DC: American Psychiatric Association, 1986), 250.

50. Richard McNally, *Remembering Trauma* (Cambridge, MA: Belknap Press of Harvard University Press, 2003), 5.

51. *DSM-III*, 259.

52. *DSM-III*, 258.

53. Hacking, *Rewriting the Soul*, 33.

54. *DSM-III-R*, 271.

55. Frank W. Putnam, *Diagnosis and Treatment of Multiple Personality Disorder* (New York: Guilford Press, 1989), 297.

56. *DSM-III-R*, 271.

57. Winter, *Memory*, 227.

58. While the hysterics that Charcot and others studied and treated were depicted in photographs that became well known in the culture at large, at the time the media was limited to printed material. By the 1980s, television, film, and mass market publishing had an exponentially greater ability to distribute models of stereotypically traumatized patients to the general public.

59. Showalter, *Hystories*, 166.

60. Lawrence Wright, *Remembering Satan: A Tragic Case of Recovered Memory* (New York: Vintage, 1994).

61. Ofshe and Watters, *Making Monsters*, 172.

62. Terr, *Unchained Memories*; Ofshe and Watters, *Making Monsters*, 254.

63. Ofshe and Watters, *Making Monsters*, 260.

64. Interestingly, in 1897 Freud also mentioned satanic ritual abuse as tied to some cases of hysteria. See Frederick Crews, *Freud: The Making of an Illusion* (New York: Henry Holt, 2017), 503.

65. Wright, *Remembering Satan*, 80.

66. Acocella, *Creating Hysteria*, 87.

67. Wright, *Remembering Satan*, 78.

68. Wright, *Remembering Satan*, 180. In 1999 Hammond was a coauthor of a book that received the American Psychiatric Association's highest award in law and psychiatry.

69. Wright, *Remembering Satan*, 75.

70. Daniel H. Schacter, *Searching for Memory: The Brain, the Mind, and the Past* (New York: Basic Books, 1996), 125.

71. See https://en.wikipedia.org/wiki/Wee_Care_Nursery_School_abuse _trial, retrieved July 7, 2017.

72. Schacter, *Searching for Memory*, 252.

73. Bass and Davis, *Courage to Heal*, 522.

74. Elke Geraerts, "Posttraumatic Memory," in *Clinician's Guide to Posttraumatic Stress Disorder*, ed. Gerald M. Rosen and B. Christopher Frueh (New York: John Wiley & Sons, 2010), 77–96, 84.

75. Quoted in Crews, *Memory Wars*, 65.

76. Mikkel Borch-Jacobsen, "Sybil: The Making of a Disease," *New York Review of Books*, April 24, 1997; Acocella, *Creating Hysteria*, 55–60.

77. Ofshe and Watters, *Making Monsters*, 207.

78. Acocella, *Creating Hysteria*, 8.

79. Winter, *Memory*, 44.

80. Schacter, *Searching for Memory*, 242.

81. Lenore Terr, "Childhood Traumas: An Outline and Overview," *American Journal of Psychiatry* 148 (1991): 10–20.

82. Acocella, *Creating Hysteria*, 74.

83. Schacter, *Searching for Memory*, 256.

84. E.g., Lawrence L. Langer, *Holocaust Testimonies: The Ruins of Memory* (New Haven, CT: Yale University Press, 1991); Mark Pendergrast, *Victims of Memory: Incest Accusations and Shattered Lives*, rev. ed. (London: Harper Collins, 1999).

85. Willem A. Wagenaar and Jop Groeneweg, "The Memory of Concentration Camp Survivors," *Applied Cognitive Psychology* 4 (1990): 77–87, 80.

86. McNally, *Remembering Trauma*, 125; Schacter, *Searching for Memory*, 245.

87. Bessel van der Kolk, Robert Blitz, Winthrop Burr, Sally Sherry, and Ernest Hartmann, "Nightmares and Trauma," *American Journal of Psychiatry* 141 (1994): 187–190, 188.

88. Geraerts, "Posttraumatic Memory," in Rosen and Frueh, *Clinician's Guide*, 83 (see n84).

89. McNally, *Remembering Trauma*, 275. The oft-cited statistics from Russell's surveys mentioned above stemmed from subjects who did not forget their abuse.

90. Schacter, *Searching for Memory*, 76.

91. Schacter, *Searching for Memory*, 5.

92. Schacter, *Searching for Memory*, 71.

93. Geraerts, "Posttraumatic Memory," in Rosen and Frueh, *Clinician's Guide*, 90.

94. Schacter, *Searching for Memory*, 106.

95. Sigmund Freud, "Heredity and the Aetiology of the Neuroses," in Sigmund Freud, *Collected Papers*, ed. James Strachey, trans. Joan Riviere (New York: Basic Books, 1959), 24–41.

96. Schacter, *Searching for Memory*, 269.

97. McNally, *Remembering Trauma*, 177.

98. Elizabeth Loftus and Katherine Ketcham, *Witness for the Defense: The Accused, the Eyewitnesses, and the Expert* (New York: St. Martin's Press, 1991), 20.

99. Elizabeth F. Loftus and Jacqueline E. Pickrell, "The Formation of False Memories," *Psychiatric Annals* 25 (1995): 720–725.

100. See Geraerts, "Posttraumatic Memories," in Rosen and Frueh, *Clinician's Guide*; Steven Jay Lynn, Timothy Lock, Elizabeth F. Loftus, Elisa Krackow, and Scott O. Lilienfeld, "The Remembrance of Things Past," in *Science and Pseudoscience in Clinical Psychology*, ed. S. O. Lilienfeld, S. J. Lynn, and J. M. Mohr (New York: Guilford Press, 2003), 205–239.

101. Schacter, *Searching for Memory*, 272–273.

102. Herman, *Trauma and Recovery*, 245, 247.

103. Quoted in Ofshe and Watters, *Making Monsters*, 30.

104. Terr, *Unchained Memories*, 52.

105. Winter, *Memory*, chap. 10.

106. Ofshe and Watters, *Making Monsters*.

107. Cynthia Hansen, "Dangerous Therapy: The Story of Patricia Burgus and Multiple Personality Disorder," *Chicago Magazine*, June 1, 1998.

108. Acocella, *Creating Hysteria*, 103.

109. American Psychiatric Association, *Diagnostic and Statistical Manual of Mental Disorders*, 4th ed. (Washington, DC: American Psychiatric Association, 1994), 484.

110. McHugh, *Try to Remember*, 178, 182.

111. Acocella, *Creating Hysteria*, 25.

112. Winter, *Memory*, 252.

Chapter 6. PTSD Becomes Ubiquitous

1. Philip Rieff, *The Triumph of the Therapeutic: Uses of Faith after Freud* (New York: Harper & Row, 1966).

2. Ralph Swindle, Kenneth Heller, Bernice Pescosolido, and Saeko Kikuzawa, "Responses to Nervous Breakdowns in America over a 40-Year Period," *American Psychologist* 55 (2000): 740–749. Between 1948 and 1976 the membership of the American Psychiatric Association grew more than fivefold, from less than 5,000 to more than 27,000. Nathan G. Hale Jr., *The Rise and Crisis of Psychoanalysis in the United States: Freud and the Americans, 1917–1985* (New York: Oxford University Press, 1995), 246.

3. Center for Mental Health Statistics, *Mental Health, United States, 1998* (Washington, DC: US Government Printing Office, 1998), 149.

4. David Mechanic, Donna D. McAlpine, and David A. Rochefort, *Mental Health and Social Policy*, 6th ed. (Boston: Pearson, 2014), 221.

5. E.g., Claudia Avina and William O'Donohue, "Sexual Harassment and PTSD: Is Sexual Harassment Diagnosable Trauma?," *Journal of Traumatic Stress* 15 (2002): 69–75; Frank M. Dattilio, "Extramarital Affairs," *Behavioral Therapist* 27 (2004): 76–78; Richard J. McNally, "Can We Fix PTSD in DSM-V?," *Depression and Anxiety* 26 (2009): 597–600, 598; Paul Lees-Haley, J. Randall Price, Christopher W. Williams, and Brian P. Betz, "Use of the Impact of Events Scale in the Assessment of Emotional Distress

and PTSD May Produce Misleading Results," *Journal of Forensic Neuropsychology* 2 (2001): 45–52.

6. David Morris, *The Evil Hours: A Biography of Post-Traumatic Stress Disorder* (Boston: Houghton Mifflin Harcourt, 2015), 2.

7. Allan Young, "9/11: Mental Health in the Wake of Terrorist Attacks," *Journal of Nervous and Mental Diseases* 195 (2007): 1030–1032, 1031.

8. Jeet Heer, "Stress Test," *New Republic*, June 2015, 29.

9. Richard Delgado and Jean Stefancic, *Understanding Words That Wound* (Boulder, CO: Westview Press, 2004), 13–15. Similarly, a prominent anthropologist claims that "words can be like rape—they can destroy you." Quoted in Thomas Fuller, "Let Right-Wing Speakers Come to Berkeley? Faculty Is Divided," *New York Times*, September 24, 2017, A16.

10. Nick Haslam, "Concept Creep: Psychology's Expanding Concepts of Harm and Pathology," *Psychological Inquiry* 27 (2016): 1–17.

11. Rebecca Solnit, "From Lying to Leering," *London Review of Books*, January 19, 2017, 3.

12. Allan V. Horwitz and Jerome C. Wakefield, *All We Have to Fear* (New York: Oxford University Press, 2012), 176.

13. According to Google Ngram, use of the term "trauma" itself grew 300 percent between 1960 and 2000.

14. See http://govcentral.monster.com/careers/articles/402, retrieved September 19, 2017.

15. American Psychiatric Association, *Diagnostic and Statistical Manual of Mental Disorders*, 4th ed. (Washington, DC: American Psychiatric Association, 1994), 427–428.

16. A number of peer-reviewed journal articles reported that watching television led people to develop PTSD. Gerald M. Rosen, B. Christopher Frueh, Jon D. Elhai, Anouk L. Grubagh, and Julian D. Ford, "Posttraumatic Stress Disorder and General Stress Studies," in *Clinician's Guide to Posttraumatic Stress Disorder*, ed. Gerald M. Rosen and B. Christopher Frueh (New York: John Wiley & Sons, 2010), 3–32, 19.

17. The *DSM-IV* significantly broadened the category of traumatic mental illnesses in a third way by introducing the category of acute stress disorder (ASD). This new diagnosis covered people whose symptoms developed immediately after the traumatic event and so would not qualify for a diagnosis of PTSD until a month had passed. The ASD criteria, which use the same stressor measures as PTSD, only required that dissociative, reexperience, avoidance, and arousal symptoms last for two days or more after the trauma, so even very brief responses would qualify as mental disorders. Moreover, the criteria stipulated that reactions disappearing within a month of the trauma still qualified as mental disorders. Thus, the *DSM-IV* regarded even extremely brief and transient symptoms as pathological. The

DSM-5 left the category of acute stress disorder unchanged, although it now required a three- instead of a two-day duration. American Psychiatric Association, *Diagnostic and Statistical Manual of Mental Disorders*, 5th ed. (Washington, DC: American Psychiatric Association, 2013), 280–281.

18. *DSM-5*, 271. The manual kept intact the symptom criteria of intrusive symptoms and avoidance of traumatic stimuli, splitting the earlier category of arousal into two categories: negative cognitions and mood and arousal. It also abandoned the distinction between acute and chronic PTSD in favor of a single duration lasting at least one month. In addition, it added a dissociative subtype and a subtype for children under six years old. Finally, the criteria added a category of delayed expression, in which symptoms arose six or more months after the traumatic experience.

19. E.g., Tanya M. Luhrmann, *Of Two Minds: The Growing Disorder in American Psychiatry* (New York: Alfred A. Knopf, 2000), 158–202; Allan V. Horwitz, *Creating Mental Illness* (Chicago: University of Chicago Press, 2002), 132–157; Daniel G. Blazer, *The Age of Melancholy: Major Depression and Its Social Origins* (New York: Routledge, 2005), 77–93.

20. Marilyn L. Bowman and Rachel Yehuda, "Risk Factors and the Adversity Stress Model," in *Posttraumatic Stress Disorder: Issues and Controversies*, ed. G. M. Rosen (New York: Wiley, 2008), 15–38, 28.

21. Richard McNally, *Remembering Trauma* (Cambridge, MA: Belknap Press of Harvard University Press, 2003), 280.

22. Morris, *Evil Hours*, 304.

23. Jonathan D. Moreno, *Mind Wars: Brain Science and the Military in the Twenty-First Century* (New York: Bellevue Literary Press, 2012), 154.

24. Alison Winter, *Memory: Fragments of a Modern History* (Chicago: University of Chicago Press, 2012), 262; Casey Schwartz, *In the Mind Fields: Exploring the New Science of Neuropsychoanalysis* (New York: Pantheon, 2015), 26.

25. See https://www.theatlantic.com/education/archive/2017/09/the-bad -science-behind-campus-response-to-sexual-assault/539211/, retrieved September 14, 2017.

26. Morris, *Evil Hours*, 157. The increasing attention paid to traumatic brain injury (TBI) after 2007 also bolstered the neuroscientific project; while some 1,200 TBI cases were diagnosed in 2006, in the following year 3,000 cases were reported. Because the symptoms of TBI are self-reported and subjective and perhaps another way of saying "concussion," it is often difficult to know how they differ from PTSD. Jerry Lembcke, *PTSD: Diagnosis and Identity in Post-empire America* (New York: Lexington, 2013), 142.

27. Naomi Breslau, Glenn C. Davis, Patricia Andreski, and Edward Peterson, "Traumatic Events and Post-traumatic Stress Disorder in an Ur-

ban Population of Young Adults, *Archives of General Psychiatry* 48 (1991): 216–222.

28. Ronald C. Kessler, Amanda Sonnega, Evelyn Bromet, Michael Hughes, and Christopher B. Nelson, "Posttraumatic Stress Disorder in the National Comorbidity Survey," *Archives of General Psychiatry* 52 (1995): 1048–1060.

29. Naomi Breslau and Ronald C. Kessler, "The Stressor Criterion in DSM-IV Posttraumatic Stress Disorder," *Biological Psychiatry* 50 (2001): 699–704, 703.

30. Of note was the finding that only one out of ninety-three cases of PTSD had a delayed onset; those who suffered traumas developed symptoms immediately afterward. Breslau et al., "Traumatic Events and Posttraumatic Stress Disorder."

31. Allan Young, *The Harmony of Illusions: Inventing Post-traumatic Stress Disorder* (Princeton, NJ: Princeton University Press, 1995), 130.

32. Kessler et al., "Posttraumatic Stress Disorder" (see n28).

33. Naomi Breslau, Howard D. Chilcoat, Ronald C. Kessler, and Glenn C. Davis, "Previous Exposure to Trauma and PTSD Effects of Subsequent Trauma," *American Journal of Psychiatry* 156 (1999): 902–907.

34. Elizabeth A. Hembree and Edna B. Foa, "Cognitive Behavioral Treatments for PTSD," in Rosen and Frueh, *Clinician's Guide*, 177–203, 178–179 (see n16).

35. Ben Shephard, *A War of Nerves: Soldiers and Psychiatrists in the Twentieth Century* (Cambridge, MA: Harvard University Press, 2000), 178.

36. S. J. Rachman, *Fear and Courage*, 2nd ed. (New York: W. H. Freeman, 1990), 20.

37. Shephard, *War of Nerves*, 180. Similarly, morale also rose among German civilians in heavily bombed cities.

38. Lars Weisaeth, "The History of Psychic Trauma," in *Handbook of PTSD*, 2nd ed., ed. Matthew J. Friedman, Terence M. Keane, and Patricia A. Resick Friedman (New York: Guilford, 2015), 38–59, 53.

39. Rebecca Solnit, *A Paradise Built in Hell* (New York: Viking, 2009), 8. Two major exceptions that did focus on the psychological impacts of disasters involved the aftermaths of the Coconut Grove nightclub fire in 1942 and an unexpected, devastating flood in Buffalo Creek, West Virginia, in 1972; A. Adler, "Neuropsychiatric Complications in Victims of Boston's Coconut Grove Disaster," *JAMA* 123 (1943): 1098–1101; Kai Erickson, *Everything in Its Path: Destruction of Community in the Buffalo Creek Flood* (New York: Simon & Schuster, 1978).

40. Yuval Neria, Arijit Nandi, and Sandro Galea, "Post-traumatic Stress Disorders Following Disasters: A Systematic Review," *Psychological Medicine* 38 (2008): 467–480.

41. This review concluded that between 30 and 40 percent of direct

victims, between 10 and 20 percent of rescue workers, and between 5 and 10 percent of the general population suffered from PTSD in the first year after a disaster.

42. Fran H. Norris, Matthew J. Friedman, Patricia J. Watson, Christopher M. Byrne, Eolia Diaz, and Krzysztof Kaniasty, "60,000 Disaster Victims Speak: Part I: An Empirical Review of the Empirical Literature, 1981–2001," *Psychiatry: Interpersonal and Biological Processes* 65 (2002): 207–239, 223.

43. Sandro Galea, Arijit Nandi, and David Vlahov, "The Epidemiology of Post-Traumatic Stress Disorder after Disasters," *Epidemiologic Reviews* 27 (2005): 78–91. E.g., while 54 percent of college basketball players who were involved in a crash-landing of an aircraft suffered from PTSD after one month, only 10–15 percent still reported the condition a year later. Norris et al., "60,000 Disaster Victims," 224.

44. Norris et al., "60,000 Disaster Victims," 238.

45. Solnit, *Paradise Built in Hell*, 219.

46. Cited in Richard Gist and Grant J. Devilly, "Early Intervention in the Aftermath of Trauma," in Rosen and Frueh, *Clinician's Guide*, 153–175, 156.

47. Quoted in Melvin Konner, "Trauma, Adaptation, and Resilience," in *Understanding Trauma*, ed. Laurence J. Kirmayer, Robert Lemelson, and Mark Barad (New York: Cambridge University Press, 2007), 300–338, 313.

48. James Nininger, "Letter to the Editor," *New York Times*, September 30, 2001.

49. Janet Heinrich, "Health Effects in the Aftermath of the World Trade Center Attacks. Testimony before the Subcommittee on National Security, Emerging Threats, and International Relations, Committee on Government Reform, House of Representatives, September 8, 2004," Serial No. 108–283 (Washington, DC: US Government Printing Office, 2004), 37–66.

50. Andrew J. Morris, "Psychic Aftershocks: Crisis Counseling and Disaster Relief Policy," *History of Psychology* 14 (2011): 264–286, 265.

51. Mark A. Schuster, Bradley D. Stein, Lisa H. Jaycox, Rebecca L. Collins, Grant N. Marshall, Marc N. Elliott, Annie J. Zhou, David E. Kanouse, Janina L. Morrison, and Sandra H. Berry, "A National Survey of Stress Reactions after the September 11, 2001, Terrorist Attacks," *New England Journal of Medicine* 345 (2001): 1507–1512, 1512.

52. Sandro Galea, David Vlahov, Heidi Resnick, Jennifer Ahern, Ezra Susser, Joel Gold, Michael Bucuvalas, and Dean Kilpatrick, "Trends of Probable Post-traumatic Stress Disorder in New York City after the September 11 Terrorist Attacks," *American Journal of Epidemiology* 158 (2003): 514–524.

53. Gist and Devilly, "Early Intervention," in Rosen and Frueh, *Clinician's Guide*, 164.

54. William E. Schlenger, Juesta M. Caddell, Lori Ebert, B. Kathleen Jordan, Kathryn M. Rourke, David Wilson, Lisa Thalji, J. Michael Dennis, John A. Fairbank, and Richard A. Kulka, "Psychological Reactions to Terrorist Attacks: Findings from the National Study of Americans' Reactions to September 11," *JAMA* 288 (2002): 581–588.

55. Sebastian Junger, *Tribe: On Homecoming and Belonging* (New York: Hachette Book Group, 2016), 116.

56. Richard J. McNally, Richard A. Bryant, and Anke Ehlers, "Does Early Psychological Intervention Promote Recovery from Posttraumatic Stress?," *Psychological Science in the Public Interest* 4 (2003): 45–79, 49.

57. Joseph A. Boscarino, Sandro Galea, Richard E. Adams, Jennifer Ahern, Heidi Resnick, and David Vlahov, "Utilization of Mental Health Services Following the September 11th Terrorist Attacks in Manhattan, New York City," *International Journal of Emergency Mental Health* 4 (2002): 143–156.

58. Sally Satel, "The Mental Health Crisis That Wasn't," *Psychiatric Services* 54 (2003): 1571.

59. Morris, "Psychic Aftershocks," 265.

60. Morris, "Psychic Aftershocks," 265. An example is the claim of a New Orleans psychotherapist that Hurricane Harvey, which struck Texas in 2017, triggered her PTSD because it revived memories of living through another hurricane fifty-six years earlier: "I was immediately back there, in that scene. It was like watching a movie screen," she asserted. John Schwartz and Campbell Robertson, "New Orleans Looks to Houston, and Sees Itself," *New York Times*, August 29, 2017, A14.

61. Naomi Breslau and Glenn C. Davis, "Posttraumatic Stress Disorder: The Stressor Criterion," *Journal of Nervous and Mental Disease* 175 (1987): 255–264, 262.

62. Richard A. Kulka, William E. Schlenger, John A. Fairbank, Richard L. Hough, B. Kathleen Jordan, Charles R. Marmar, and Daniel S. Weiss, *Contractual Report of the National Vietnam Veterans Readjustment Study: Executive Summary, Descriptive Findings, and Technical Appendices* (Research Triangle Park, NC: Research Triangle Institute, 1988).

63. Junger, *Tribe*, 97.

64. Shephard, *War of Nerves*, 392.

65. Robert H. Fleming, "Post Vietnam Syndrome: Neurosis or Sociosis?," *Psychiatry* 48 (1985): 122–139, 131.

66. David H. Marlowe, *Psychological and Psychosocial Consequences of Combat and Deployment* (Santa Monica, CA: Rand, 2000), 76.

67. Bruce P. Dohrenwend, J. Blake Turner, Nicholas A. Turse, Ben G. Adams, Karestan C. Koenen, and Randall Marshall, "The Psychological Risks of Vietnam for U.S. Veterans: A Revisit with New Data and Methods," *Science* 313 (2006): 979–982.

68. Richard J. McNally. "Revisiting Dohrenwend et al.'s Revisit of the National Vietnam Veterans Readjustment Study," *Journal of Traumatic Stress* 20 (2007): 481–486, 483.

69. Richard J. McNally and B. Christopher Frueh, "Why Are Iraq and Afghanistan War Veterans Seeking PTSD Disability Compensation at Unprecedented Rates?," *Journal of Anxiety Disorders* 27 (2013): 520–526, 521.

70. Hans Pols and Stephanie Oak, "War and Military Mental Health," *American Journal of Public Health* 97 (2007): 2132–2142.

71. Department of Defense, "PostTraumatic Stress Disorder and Traumatic Brain Injury Research Program," http://cdmrp.army.mil/pubs/press /2007/07ptsdtbipreann.htm accessed, September 17, 2017.

72. Bryan Doerries, *The Theater of War: What Ancient Greek Tragedies Can Teach Us Today* (New York: Knopf, 2015), 117.

73. E.g., Charles W. Hoge, Carl A. Castro, Stephen C. Messer, Dennis McGurk, Dave I. Cotting, and Robert L. Koffman, "Combat Duty in Iraq and Afghanistan, Mental Health Problems, and Barriers to Care," *New England Journal of Medicine* 351 (2004): 13–22.

74. Jessica Wolfe, Darin J. Erickson, Erica J. Sharkansky, Daniel W. King, and Dynda A. King, "Course and Predictors of Posttraumatic Stress Disorder among Gulf War Veterans: A Prospective Analysis," *Journal of Counseling and Clinical Psychology* 67 (1999): 520–528.

75. Hoge et al., "Combat Duty in Iraq and Afghanistan"; Charles W. Hoge, Jennifer L. Auchterlonie, and Charles S. Milliken, "Mental Health Problems, Use of Mental Health Services, and Attrition from Military Service after Returning from Deployment to Iraq or Afghanistan," *JAMA* 295 (2007): 1023–1032. Military researchers claim that even drone operators who are thousands of miles away from combat zones now develop rates of PTSD at rates as high as flyers in combat. James Dao, "Drone Pilots Are Found to Get Stress Disorders Much as Those in Combat Do," *New York Times*, February 22, 2013.

76. Karen H. Seal, Daniel Bertenthal, Christian Miner, Saunak Sen, and Charles Marmar, "Bringing the War Back Home: Mental Health Disorders among 103,788 US Veterans Returning from Iraq and Afghanistan Seen at Department of Veterans Affairs Facilities," *Archives of Internal Medicine* 167 (2007): 476–482.

77. Seal et al., "Bringing the War Back Home."

78. American Psychological Association, *The Psychological Needs of U.S. Military Service Members and Their Families* (Washington, DC: American Psychological Association, 2007), 26.

79. Hoge et al., "Combat Duty in Iraq and Afghanistan," 19.

80. Department of the Army, *Army Health Promotion/Risk Reduction/*

Suicide Prevention Report 2010 (Washington, DC: Department of the Army, 2010); Kenneth T. MacLeish, *Making War at Fort Hood* (Princeton, NJ: Princeton University Press, 2013), 226.

81. Doerries, *Theater of War*, 97.

82. Matthew J. Friedman, "Suicide Risk among Soldiers," *JAMA Psychiatry* 71 (2014): 487–489, 488.

83. MacLeish, *Making War at Fort Hood*, 112.

84. Lembcke, *PTSD*, 24.

85. Institute of Medicine, *Returning Home from Iraq and Afghanistan: Assessment of Readjustment Needs of Veterans, Service Members, and Their Families* (Washington, DC: National Academies Press, 2013).

86. Daniel M. Gade, "A Better Way to Help Veterans," *National Affairs* 16 (2013): 53–69.

87. Rand Corporation, "One in Five Iraq or Afghanistan Veterans Suffer from PTSD or Major Depression," http://www.rand.org/news/press /2008/04/17.html, accessed September 17, 2017.

88. Morris, *Evil Hours*, 161.

89. MacLeish, *Making War at Fort Hood*, 4. David Morris claims that alcohol is the best PTSD drug ever invented (*Evil Hours*, 229).

90. Beth E. Cohen, Ying Shi, Thomas C. Neylan, Shira Maguen, and Karen H. Seal, "Antipsychotic Prescriptions in Iraq and Afghanistan Veterans with Posttraumatic Stress Disorder in Department of Veterans Affairs Healthcare, 2007–2012," *Journal of Clinical Psychiatry* 76 (2015): 406–412.

91. Morris, *Evil Hours*, 177–190.

92. Elizabeth A. Hembree and Edna B. Foa, "Cognitive Behavioral Treatments for PTSD," in Rosen and Frueh, *Clinician's Guide*, 177–203, 186; McNally, *Remembering Trauma*, 187.

93. Winter, *Memory*, 266.

94. Jeneen Interlandi, "How Do You Heal a Traumatized Mind?," *New York Times Sunday Magazine*, May 25, 2014, MM42.

95. Dave Phillips, "Scuba, Parrots, Yoga: Many Veterans Embrace Alternative Therapies for PTSD," *New York Times*, September 18, 2016, A12.

96. Bret A. Moore and Walter E. Penk, *Treating PTSD in Military Personnel: A Clinical Handbook* (New York: Guilford, 2011).

97. Simon Wessely, "War and the Mind: Suffering or Psychopathology," *Palestine-Israeli Journal of Politics, Economics, and Culture* 10, see http:// www.pij.org/details.php?id=55, accessed September 17, 2017.

98. McHugh, *Try to Remember*, 194.

99. Institute of Medicine, *Treatment of Posttraumatic Stress Disorder: An Assessment of the Evidence* (Washington, DC: National Academies Press, 2008).

100. "Interest [in such treatments] has just exploded," one VA psychiatrist explained. "There is no one who thinks this is just silly alternative medicine stuff anymore." Phillips, "Scuba, Parrots, Yoga," A12.

101. McNally, Bryant, and Ehlers, "Early Psychological Intervention."

102. Mental Health Advisory Team, *Operation Iraqi Freedom* (Washington, DC: Office of the Surgeon General, 2009).

103. McHugh, *Try to Remember*, 189.

104. Interlandi, "How Do You Heal?," 42.

105. Charles W. Hoge, "Interventions for War-related Posttraumatic Stress Disorder: Meeting Veterans Where They Are," *JAMA* 306 (2011): 549–551.

106. MacLeish, *Making War at Fort Hood*, 52, 94, 118, 120, 123–124.

107. MacLeish, *Making War at Fort Hood*, 124.

108. Morris, *Evil Hours*, 261.

109. Erin Finley, *Fields of Combat: Understanding PTSD among Veterans of Iraq and Afghanistan* (Ithaca, NY: IRL Press), 130.

110. MacLeish, *Making War at Fort Hood*, 120–123.

111. McNally and Frueh, "Iraq and Afghanistan War Veterans."

112. Alan Zarembo, "As Disability Awards Grow, So Do Concerns with Veracity of PTSD Claims," *Los Angeles Times*, August 3, 2014.

113. McNally and Frueh, "Iraq and Afghanistan War Veterans," 520.

114. Matthew Hotopf, Lisa Hull, Nicola T. Fear, Tess Browne, Oded Horn, Amy Iverson, Margaret Jones, Dominic Murphy, Duncan Bland, Mark Earnshaw, Neil Greenberg, Jamie H. Hughes, A. Rosemary Tate, Christopher Dandeker, Roberto Rona, and Simon Wessely, "The Health of UK Military Personnel Who Deployed to the 2003 Iraq War," *Lancet* 367 (2006): 1731–1741; Mark A. Turner, Mathew Kiernan, Andrew G. Mc-Kechanie, Peter J. Finch, Frank B. McManus, and Leigh A. Neal, "Acute Military Psychiatric Casualties from the War in Iraq," *British Journal of Psychiatry* 186 (2005): 476–479.

115. Robert A. Rosenheck and Alan F. Fontana, "Recent Trends in VA Treatment of Post-Traumatic Stress Disorder and Other Mental Disorders," *Health Affairs* 26 (2007): 1720–1727.

116. Richard J. McNally, "Psychiatric Casualties of War," *Science* 313 (2006): 923–924, 923.

117. Gerald M. Rosen and Steven Taylor, "Pseudo-PTSD," *Journal of Anxiety Disorders* 21 (2007): 201–210, 202.

118. Zarembo, "As Disability Awards Grow."

119. Charles W. Hoge, Herb Goldberg, and Carl Castro, "Care of War Veterans with Mild Traumatic Brain Injury—Flawed Perspectives," *New England Journal of Medicine* 360 (2009): 588–591.

120. B. Christopher Frueh, Mark B. Hamner, Shawn P. Cahill, Paul B.

Gold, and Kasey L. Hamlin, "Apparent Symptom Overreporting in Combat Veterans Evaluated for PTSD," *Clinical Psychology Review* 20 (2000): 853–884, 865.

121. B. Christopher Frueh, Jon D. Elhai, Paul B. Gold, Jeannine Monnier, Kathryn M. Magruder, Terence M. Keane, and George W. Arana, "Disability Compensation Seeking among Veterans Evaluated for Posttraumatic Stress Disorder," *Psychiatric Services* 54 (2003): 84–91.

122. Joshua D. Angrist, Stacey H. Chen, and Brigham R. Frandsen, "Did Vietnam Veterans Get Sicker in the 1990s? The Complicated Effects of Military Service on Self-Reported Health," *Journal of Public Economics* 94 (2010): 824–837; David H. Autor, Mark G. Duggan, and David S. Lyle, "Battle Scars? The Puzzling Decline in Employment and Rise in Disability Receipt among Vietnam Era Veterans," *American Economic Review* 101 (2011): 339–344; Jason Schnittker, *The Diagnostic System* (New York: Columbia University Press, 2017), 232.

123. B. Christopher Frueh, Anouk L. Grubaugh, Jon D. Elhai, and Todd C. Buckley, "US Department of Veterans Affairs Disability Policies for Posttraumatic Stress Disorder," *American Journal of Public Health* 97 (2007): 3143–3150.

124. Alan Zarembo, "As Disability Awards Grow, So Do Concerns with Veracity of PTSD Claims," *Los Angeles Times*, August 3, 2014.

125. Shankar Vedantam, "VA Benefits System for PTSD Victims Is Criticized," *Washington Post*, May 9, 2007.

126. Thomas Freeman, Melissa Powell, and Tim Kimbrell, "Measuring Symptom Exaggeration in Veterans with Chronic Posttraumatic Stress Disorder," *Psychiatry Research* 158 (2008): 374–380.

127. B. Christopher Frueh, Jon D. Elhai, Anouk L. Grubaugh, Jeannine Monnier, Todd B. Kashdan, Julie A. Sauvageot, Mark B. Hamner, B. G. Burkett, and George W. Arana, "Documented Combat Exposure of US Veterans Seeking Treatment for Combat-Related Post-traumatic Stress Disorder," *British Journal of Psychiatry* 186 (2005): 467–472.

128. Frueh et al., "Apparent Symptom Overreporting"; Steven M. Southwick, C. Andrew Morgan, Andreas L. Nicolaou, and Dennis Charney, "Consistency of Memory for Combat-Related Traumatic Events in Veterans of Operation Desert Storm," *American Journal of Psychiatry* 154 (1997): 173–177, 174.

129. Vedantam, "VA Benefits System."

130. Zarembo, "As Disability Awards Grow."

131. Quoted in Finley, *Fields of Combat*, 116.

132. Finley, *Fields of Combat*, 127.

133. Allan V. Horwitz and Jerome C. Wakefield, *The Loss of Sadness: Psychiatry's Transformation of Normal Sadness into Depressive Disorder* (New

York: Oxford University Press, 2007); Horwitz and Wakefield, *All We Have to Fear*.

134. Willard W. Waller, *The Veteran Comes Back* (1944; San Francisco: Forgotten Books, 2006), 189.

135. Didier Fassin and Richard Rechtman, *The Empire of Trauma* (Princeton, NJ: Princeton University Press, 2009).

136. David Rieff, *In Praise of Forgetting: Historical Memory and Its Ironies* (New Haven, CT: Yale University Press, 2016), 144.

Chapter 7. Implications

1. American Psychiatric Association, *Diagnostic and Statistical Manual of Mental Disorders*, 5th ed. (Washington, DC: American Psychiatric Association, 2013), 271–272.

2. Charles Rosenberg, *Our Present Complaint: American Medicine Then and Now* (Baltimore: Johns Hopkins University Press, 2007), 13.

3. Robert L. Spitzer, Michael B. First, and Jerome C. Wakefield, "Saving PTSD from Itself in DSM-V," *Journal of Anxiety Disorders* 21 (2007): 233–241.

4. Allan V. Horwitz, *Creating Mental Illness* (Chicago: University of Chicago Press, 2002).

5. Mark S. Micale, "Jean-Martin Charcot and *les neuroses traumatiques*," in *Traumatic Pasts: History, Psychiatry, and Trauma in the Modern Age, 1870–1930*, ed. Mark S. Micale and Paul Lerner (New York: Cambridge University Press, 2001), 115–139, 122.

6. Sigmund Freud, "Heredity and the Aetiology of the Neuroses," in Sigmund Freud, *Collected Papers*, trans. Joan Riviere (New York: Basic Books, 1959), 138–154, 149.

7. Ralph Harrington, "The Railway Accident," in Micale and Lerner, *Traumatic Pasts*, 31–56 (see n5).

8. Sigmund Freud, *Beyond the Pleasure Principle*, trans. James Strachey (New York: W. W. Norton, 1989).

9. Quoted in Didier Fassin and Richard Rechtman, *The Empire of Trauma* (Princeton, NJ: Princeton University Press, 2009), 61.

10. Edgar Jones and Simon Wessely, *Shell Shock to PTSD: Military Psychiatry from 1900 to the Gulf War* (New York: Psychology Press, 2005), 57.

11. Quoted in Allan Young, *The Harmony of Illusions: Inventing Post-Traumatic Stress Disorder* (Princeton, NJ: Princeton University Press, 1995), 54.

12. Gerald N. Grob, *From Asylum to Community: Mental Health Policy in Modern America* (Princeton, NJ: Princeton University Press, 1991), 12.

13. American Psychological Association, *Diagnostic and Statistical Manual of Mental Disorders*, 3rd ed. (Washington, DC: American Psychiatric Association, 1980), 238.

14. Chaim F. Shatan, "Have You Hugged a Vietnam Veteran Today? The Basic Wound of Catastrophic Stress," in *Post-Traumatic Stress Disorder and the War Veteran Patient*, ed. W. E. Kelly (New York: Brunner/Mazel, 1985), 12–28, 21.

15. Ben Shephard, *A War of Nerves: Soldiers and Psychiatrists in the Twentieth Century* (Cambridge, MA: Harvard University Press, 2000), 391; Marilyn L. Bowman and Rachel Yehuda, "Risk Factors and the Adversity Stress Model," in *Posttraumatic Stress Disorder: Issues and Controversies*, ed. G. M. Rosen (New York: Wiley, 2008), 15–38.

16. American Psychiatric Association, *Diagnostic and Statistical Manual of Mental Disorders*, 4th ed. (Washington, DC: American Psychiatric Association, 1994), 428.

17. Richard McNally, *Remembering Trauma* (Cambridge, MA: Belknap Press of Harvard University Press, 2003), 280.

18. Bowman and Yehuda, "Risk Factors," 28.

19. Southborough, 1922, quoted in Jones and Wessely, *Shell Shock to PTSD*, 54, 151. Edgar Jones, Ian Palmer, and Simon Wessely, "War Pensions (1900–1945): Changing Models of Psychological Understanding," *British Journal of Psychiatry* 180 (2002): 374–379, 376.

20. Nancy Andreasen, "Posttraumatic Stress Disorder: Psychology, Biology, and the Manichean Warfare between False Dichotomies," *American Journal of Psychiatry* 152 (1995): 964.

21. Autism provides another exception to the negative connotations of most mental illness diagnoses. Like PTSD, it entered the *DSM* primarily through the efforts of lay activists, in particular, parents of afflicted individuals. And, like PTSD, diagnoses of autism (now called "autistic spectrum disorders") provide pathways to desired resources in schools, clinical treatments, and assistance in daily living. Ian Hacking, "On the Ratio of Science to Activism in the Shaping of Autism," in *Philosophical Issues in Psychiatry III: The Nature and Sources of Historical Change*, ed. K. S. Kendler and J. Parnas (New York: Oxford University Press, 2015), 326–339.

22. Fassin and Rechtman, *Empire of Trauma*.

23. Quoted in Harrington, "Railway Accident," 55.

24. Michael R. Trimble, *Post-Traumatic Neurosis: From Railway Spine to the Whiplash* (New York: John Wiley & Sons, 1981).

25. Eric Caplan, "Trains and Trauma in the American Gilded Age," in Micale and Lerner, *Traumatic Pasts*, 57–80.

26. Shephard, *War of Nerves*.

27. While veterans' compensation has been the most prominent arena for PTSD claims, these claims also often result from accidents and other personal injuries, criminal victimizations, natural and man-made disasters, workplace harassments, and the like.

28. John M. Kinder, *Paying with Their Bodies: American War and the Problem of the Disabled Veteran* (Chicago: University of Chicago Press, 2015).

29. Shephard, *War of Nerves*, 167.

30. Sigmund Freud, "Psychoanalysis and War Neuroses," in *The Standard Edition of the Complete Psychological Works of Sigmund Freud*, ed. and trans. James Strachey (1919; London: Hogarth Press, 1955), 17:207–210, 207.

31. Abram Kardiner, *Traumatic Neuroses of War* (New York: Harper & Brothers, 1941), 211.

32. Kardiner, *Traumatic Neuroses*, 218.

33. Quoted in Fassin and Rechtman, *Empire of Trauma*, 37.

34. Quoted in Fassin and Rechtman, *Empire of Trauma*, 64, 65.

35. Greg A. Eghigian, "The German Welfare State as a Discourse of Trauma," in Micale and Lerner, *Traumatic Pasts*, 92–114, 107, 108.

36. Quoted in Fassin and Rechtman, *Empire of Trauma*, 70.

37. The diagnosis also provided a resource through which feminist therapists could attribute liability to fathers (and occasionally other relatives); many encouraged abused daughters to bring lawsuits against them. Unlike the liability of railroad companies and governments, however, the benefits from successful litigation for sexual maltreatment were usually psychic, not monetary, in nature.

38. Allan V. Horwitz and Jerome C. Wakefield, *All We Have to Fear* (New York: Oxford University Press, 2012), 185.

39. Eric T. Dean Jr., *Shook over Hell: Post-Traumatic Stress, Vietnam, and the Civil War* (Cambridge, MA: Harvard University Press, 1991), 148.

40. Sarah Haley, "When the Patient Reports Atrocities: Specific Treatment Considerations of the Vietnam Veteran," *Archives of General Psychiatry* 30 (1974): 191–196, 191. Although their identities were never known, some critics claim that many of Haley's patients were never actually at My Lai. B. G. Burkett and Glenna Whitley, *Stolen Valor: How the Vietnam Generation Was Robbed of Its Heroes and Its History* (Dallas: Verity Press, 1998), 154–158.

41. E.g., B. Christopher Frueh, Mark B. Hamner, Shawn P. Cahill, Paul B. Gold, and Kasey L. Hamlin, "Apparent Symptom Overreporting in Combat Veterans Evaluated for PTSD," *Clinical Psychology Review* 20 (2000): 853–884. "The image of the victim-veteran had become such a compelling element in the American imagination of what the return from war should be that it was evoking the very health problems that it proposed to describe," one sociologist observed. Jerry Lembcke, *PTSD: Diagnosis and Identity in Post-empire America* (New York: Lexington, 2013), 12.

42. Richard J. McNally and B. Christopher Frueh, "Why Are Iraq and Afghanistan War Veterans Seeking PTSD Disability Compensation at Unprecedented Rates?," *Journal of Anxiety Disorders* 27 (2013): 520–526. Empir-

ical studies that attempt to distinguish simulators from genuinely damaged claimants typically find that, while many claimants experienced the sorts of highly stressful conditions that bring about traumas, a substantial number did not, and a few clearly fabricated their symptoms.

43. E.g., Jones and Wessely, *Shell Shock to PTSD*; McNally, *Remembering Trauma*. As Chapter 6 noted, a major US Army report indicates that post-combat symptomology dissipates in most soldiers after twenty-four months and is indistinguishable from a control group after thirty-six months. See https://www.google.com/url?sa=t&rct=j&q=&esrc=s&source=web&cd =2&ved=0ahUKEwjn_dHfgqLVAhUIyj4KHSkjC9AQFggtMAE&url=h ttp%3A%2F%2Farmymedicine.mil%2FDocuments%2FMHAT-VI-OIF _EXSUM.pdf&usg=AFQjCNHE38xYrIN_4Uvjps5ieyUKwQC_tg&cad =rja. Accessed July 24, 2017.

44. Alan Zarembo, "As Disability Awards Grow, So Do Concerns with Veracity of PTSD Claims," *Los Angeles Times*, August 3, 2014.

45. Institute of Medicine, *Treatment of Posttraumatic Stress Disorder: An Assessment of the Evidence* (Washington, DC: National Academies Press, 2008); Christina Hoff Sommers and Sally Satel, *One Nation under Therapy* (New York: St. Martin's, 2005), 216.

46. Paul R. McHugh, "How Psychiatry Lost Its Way," *Commentary* 108 (1999): 32–38, 35.

47. Edward Shorter, *A History of Psychiatry: From the Era of Psychiatry to the Age of Prozac* (New York: John Wiley, 1997).

48. Micale, "Jean-Martin Charcot."

49. Nancy Andreasen, *Brave New Brain* (New York: Oxford University Press, 2001), 296.

50. Gerald M. Rosen, Scott O. Lilienfeld, and Scott P. Orr, "Searching for PTSD's Biological Signature," in *Clinician's Guide to Posttraumatic Stress Disorder*, ed. Gerald M. Rosen and B. Christopher Frueh (New York: John Wiley & Sons, 2010), 97–116, 110.

51. Rachel Yehuda and Alexander McFarlane, "Conflict between Current Knowledge about Posttraumatic Stress Disorder and Its Original Conceptual Basis," *American Journal of Psychiatry* 152 (1995): 1705–1713.

52. Judith Herman, *Trauma and Recovery* (New York: Basic Books, 2015), 256.

53. Rosen, Lilienfeld, and Orr, "Searching," in Micale and Lerner, *Traumatic Pasts*.

54. Institute of Medicine, *Posttraumatic Stress Disorder: Diagnosis and Assessment* (Washington, DC: National Academies Press, 2006), 46.

55. Naomi Breslau and Glenn C. Davis, "Posttraumatic Stress Disorder: The Stressor Criterion," *Journal of Nervous and Mental Disease* 175 (1987): 255–264; Rosen, Lilienfeld, and Orr, "Searching."

56. Steven E. Hyman, "The Diagnosis of Mental Disorders: The Problem of Reification," *Annual Review of Clinical Psychology* 6 (2010): 155–179. Despite the absence of reliable knowledge about the neurobiological aspects of trauma, its use is becoming more widespread in judicial proceedings involving accusation of trauma victimizations. See Emily Yoffe, "The Bad Science behind the Campus Response to Sexual Assault," https://www.the atlantic.com/education/archive/2017/09/the-bad-science-behind-campus -response-to-sexual-assault/539211/ accessed September 17, 2017.

57. Sara Reardon, "Drug Helps to Clear Traumatic Memories," *Nature News*, January 16, 2014.

58. Fassin and Rechtman, *Empire of Trauma*, 284.

59. Young, *Harmony of Illusions*.

60. Lawrence A. Tritle, "'Ravished Minds' in the Ancient World," in *Combat Trauma and the Ancient Greeks*, ed. Peter Meineck and David Konstan (New York: Palgrave Macmillan, 2014), 87–105, 96. Psychiatrist Jonathan Shay, whose readings of the *Iliad* and the *Odyssey* have been especially influential shapers of the idea that PTSD has been present in all times and places, believes that "Homer has seen things that we in psychiatry and psychology have more or less missed." Jonathan Shay, *Achilles in Vietnam: Combat Trauma and the Undoing of Character* (New York: Scribner, 1994), xiii; Jonathan Shay, *Odysseus in America: Combat Trauma and the Trials of Homecoming* (New York: Scribner, 2002). Unlike many of his followers, Shay himself does not rely on neuroscientific findings but, instead, on the universal moral responses that soldiers make to the dishonorable actions of their commanders.

61. E.g., R. J. Daly, "Samuel Pepys and Post-traumatic Stress Disorder," *British Journal of Psychiatry* 143 (1983): 64–68. Philip A. Mackowiak and Sonja Batten, "Post-Traumatic Stress Reactions before the Advent of Post Traumatic Stress Disorder: Potential Effects on the Lives and Legacies of Alexander the Great, Captain James Cook, Emily Dickinson, and Florence Nightingale," *Military Medicine* 173 (2008): 1158–1163; Lawrence A. Tritle, *From Melos to My Lai: War and Survival* (New York: Routledge, 2000); Kurt A. Raaflaub, "War and the City: The Brutality of War and Its Impact on the Community," in Meineck and Konstan, *Combat Trauma and the Ancient Greeks*, 15–46 (see n60); Bryan Doerries, *The Theater of War* (New York: Knopf, 2015); Yulia Ustinova and Etzel Cardeña, "Combat Stress Disorders and Their Treatment in Ancient Greece," *Psychological Trauma: Theory, Research, Practice, and Policy* 6 (2014): 739–748; Sharon James, "The Battered Shield: Survivor Guilt and Family Trauma in Menander's *Aspis*," in Meineck and Konstan, *Combat Trauma and the Ancient Greeks*, 237–260; S. Sara Monoson, "Socrates in Combat: Trauma and Resilience in Plato's Political

Theory," in Meineck and Konstan, *Combat Trauma and the Ancient Greeks*, 131–162.

62. Crowley, in Meineck and Konstan, *Combat Trauma and the Ancient Greeks*, 112.

63. Van Wees, "Greek Warfare," in Meineck and Konstan, *Combat Trauma and the Ancient Greeks*, 111.

64. Edward Shorter, *From Paralysis to Fatigue: A History of Psychosomatic Illness in the Modern Era* (New York: Free Press, 1992), 320.

65. J. M. Da Costa, "On Irritable Heart: A Clinical Study of a Functional Cardiac Disorder and Its Consequences, *American Journal of the Medical Sciences* 61 (1871): 17–52; Shephard, *War of Nerves*; Edgar Jones, Robert H. Vermaas, Helen McCartney, Charlotte Beech, Ian Palmer, Kenneth Hyams, and Simon Wessely, "Flashbacks and Post-Traumatic Stress Disorder: The Genesis of a Twentieth-Century Diagnosis," *British Journal of Psychiatry* 182 (2003): 158–163.

66. Rosenberg, *Our Present Complaint*, 5.

67. Jones and Wessely, *Shell Shock to PTSD*, 135.

68. Wilbur J. Scott, "PTSD in *DSM-III*: A Case in the Politics of Diagnosis and Disease," *Social Problems* 37 (1990): 294–310.

69. Fassin and Rechtman, *Empire of Trauma*.

70. E.g., Allan V. Horwitz and Jerome C. Wakefield, *The Loss of Sadness: Psychiatry's Transformation of Normal Sadness into Depressive Disorder* (New York: Oxford University Press, 2007); Horwitz and Wakefield, *All We Have to Fear*.

71. Marijuana is one potentially effective treatment for PTSD that the VA is forbidden to prescribe. See Thomas James Brennan, "Why Pot, Not Pills, Works for My T.B.I.," *New York Times*, September 1, 2017, A 23. In 2016 the Food and Drug Administration did allow drug companies to proceed with clinical trials that will test the effectiveness of the "club drug" ecstasy as a treatment for PTSD.

72. E.g., Frank Furedi, *Therapy Culture: Cultivating Vulnerability in an Uncertain Age* (New York: Routledge, 2003); Christopher Lasch, *The Culture of Narcissism* (New York: W. W. Norton, 1979); Timothy Aubry and Trysh Travis, eds., *Rethinking Therapeutic Culture* (Chicago: University of Chicago Press, 2015).

73. E.g., Chris Walsh, *Cowardice: A Brief History* (Princeton, NJ: Princeton University Press, 2014).

74. As Chapter 1 noted, the Google Ngram viewer indicates that after 1980 the use of the term "PTSD" increased by about 350 percent in the following twenty-eight years. Conversely, the use of the words "courage" and "cowardice" fell by about 400 percent from 1800 to 2000.

75. Allan Young and Naomi Breslau, "Troublesome Memories: Reflections on the Future," *Journal of Anxiety Disorders* 21 (2007): 230–232, 231.

76. See https://www.google.com/#q=fox+news+stories+on+ptsd, retrieved July 22, 2017; https://www.nytimes.com/topic/subject/veterans-and -post-traumatic-stress-disorder, retrieved July 22, 2017. https://www.ny times.com/2017/08/02/us/finding-some-peace-after-war.html?_r=0, retrieved August 3, 2017.

77. Cf. German E. Berrios, "The Role of Cultural Configurators in the Formation of Mental Symptoms," in *Philosophical Issues in Psychiatry III: The Nature and Sources of Historical Change*, ed. Kenneth S. Kendler and Josef Parnas (New York: Oxford University Press, 2015), 107–115, 114.

78. Simon Wessely, "Victimhood and Resilience," *New England Journal of Medicine* 353 (2005): 548–550, 549.

79. Bruce N. Cuthbert and Thomas R. Insel, "Toward the Future of Psychiatric Diagnosis: The Seven Pillars of RDoC," *BMC Medicine* 11 (2013): 126.

80. E.g., Sally Satel and Scott O. Lilienfeld, *Brainwashed: The Seductive Appeal of Mindless Neuroscience* (New York: Basic Books, 2015); Allen Frances, *Saving Normal: An Insider's Revolt against Out-of-Control Diagnoses* (New York: William Morrell, 2013); Rosen and Frueh, *Clinician's Guide* (see n50).

INDEX

Abraham, Karl, 57, 170
acute stress disorder (ASD), 215n17
Adams, Michael, 26
Afghanistan War, 2, 152–53, 154, 156–57, 158, 220n75
Airplane (movie), 205n29
American Legion, 66, 75–76, 87
American Psychiatric Association (APA), 92–93, 214n2
Andreasen, Nancy, 87, 97, 161, 179; on desirability of PTSD diagnosis, 10–11, 173; on PTSD symptoms, 101–2, 208n87
Apple, John, 71
Assault on Truth (Masson), 112
autism, 225n21

Babinski, Joseph, 37, 125
Barr, Roseanne, 122
Bass, Ellen, 115–16, 117, 125, 131–32
Beard, George, 193n20
Beebe, Gilbert, 71
Benedikt, Moritz, 34
Bernheim, Hippolyte, 37, 125–26
Best Years of Our Lives, The (movie), 76
Bettelheim, Bruno, 89
Beyond the Pleasure Principle (Freud), 58
Bierce, Ambrose, 26
Borch-Jacobsen, Mikkel, 16
Bourne, Peter, 86
Bowman, Marilyn, 142, 173
Bradley, Omar, 74
brain, 52, 56, 142; and mind, 13–17, 40, 178–81; scans of, 143. *See also* neuroscience
Braun, Bennett, 132
Breslau, Naomi, 149–50, 186

Breuer, Josef, 40–42, 45–47
Brissaud, Édouard, 176
Broca, Pierre Paul, 20
Brokaw, Tom, 77
Bryant, Richard, 149

Caplan, Eric, 31
Cardeña, Etzel, 14
Charcot, Jean-Martin, 17; on environmental and psychic causes, 14, 36, 179; hereditarian views of, 35, 40, 50, 52; on hysteria, 35–37, 169
childhood sexual abuse: false memories of, 125–27, 130, 132; Freud on, 42–43, 44–45, 50, 110–12, 130, 169, 210n15; media coverage of, 121–24; and recovered memory movement, 108–9, 110, 112, 115–16, 121–25; severity of, 127–28
Civil War, 49; combat during, 21–23; and veterans' compensation, 26–28; veterans' symptoms from, 23–26
Cleveland, Grover, 27
Combat Exhaustion (report), 71
"combat neurosis," 3, 63, 70, 82, 100, 141, 150, 167; military psychiatrists on, 73, 141
Coming Home (movie), 86
community treatment, 81
compensation: and Civil War pensions, 26–28; as inducement to chronic conditions, 97, 160–62, 177–78, 226n42; and liability issues, 175, 225n27; for PTSD, 157–62, 174; for "railway spine" injuries, 31–33. *See also* pensions
consciousness, two states of, 34, 37–38
Courage to Heal, The (Bass and Davis), 115–16, 117, 125

court litigation, 50, 226n37; over railroad
    crashes, 28, 32–33; and recovered mem-
    ory movement, 117, 132–33
cowardice and malingering, 13, 29, 52, 139,
    150, 182, 186, 187; Civil War view of, 21,
    22–23, 24; and compensation claims,
    32, 36, 141, 174; and DSM, 85, 139, 171;
    World War I view of, 55, 56, 60, 65, 170;
    World War II view of, 71–72, 73–74
cultural symptom pool, 182–83

Da Costa, Jacob, 24–26, 183
Davis, Glenn, 149–50
Davis, Laura, 115–16, 117, 125
Dean, Eric, 87
Deer Hunter (movie), 86
Delgado, Richard, 138
Diagnostic and Statistical Manual of
    Mental Disorders. See DSM
Dickens, Charles, 30
Disabled American Veterans of the World
    War, 66, 75–76
disasters, 146–50, 217n41, 218n43
dissociation, 128–29; Janet on, 37, 38–39,
    112–13
dissociative identity disorder (DID), 133
Donohue, Phil, 122
double consciousness, 34
dreams, 59
drug companies, 185, 229n71
drug therapies, 64, 72, 154
DSM (Diagnostic and Statistical Manual
    of Mental Disorders), 6, 139–41, 166–68,
    187–88
DSM-I, 82, 83–84
DSM-II, 84–85
DSM-III, 58, 93–98, 105–6, 138, 139, 166,
    171, 176, 184; diagnostic criteria in, 7,
    18, 98–100, 141–42; on PTSD symp-
    toms, 101–4; trauma definition in, 172
DSM-III-R, 120, 121, 139, 140, 144
DSM-IV, 139–40, 142–43, 144, 215n17
DSM-5, 140, 166, 216nn17-18
Dworkin, Andrea, 108

Ehlers, Anke, 149
Ellenberger, Henri, 16

environmental and external factors:
    DSM-III on, 103–4, 106; vs. psychic
    and hereditary predisposition, 8–10, 31,
    56–57, 70, 80–81, 101, 141–44, 168–73;
    World War II conclusions about,
    71–72, 79, 82–83, 179
Epidemiologic Catchment Area (ECA)
    research, 105
Erichsen, John, 28–29, 178–79
exposure therapy, 154–55

false memories, 125–26, 130–32
False Memory Syndrome Foundation
    (FMSF), 132
Fassin, Didier, 163, 181
Federal Emergency Management Agency
    (FEMA), 148, 149
Felix, Robert, 81
feminism, 39, 81–82, 108, 115, 209n2
Ferenczi, Sándor, 57
Finley, Erin, 157, 162
Fischer-Homberger, Esther, 56
flashbacks, 26, 87, 138, 183, 205n30,
    208n86
Fliess, Wilhelm, 48
Frederickson, Renee, 109
Freud, Sigmund, 17, 39–45; on childhood
    sexual memories, 42–43, 44, 50, 110–12,
    130, 169, 210n15; on hypnosis, 47–48;
    on hysteria, 40–41, 42, 52; impact on
    Kardiner, 59, 101; Janet criticisms of,
    38, 39, 196n100; on repressed memory,
    39, 41–42, 43–44, 52, 169, 196n100;
    seduction theory of, 44–45, 48, 111, 112;
    on traumatic neuroses, 40, 41, 42–43,
    57–59, 101, 103, 179; treatment by, 5,
    45–49, 50; on unconscious, 42–43, 50,
    59; on war trauma, 57–58, 102, 169–70,
    175–76, 199n21
Frueh, Christopher, 160–61

Gall, Franz Joseph, 20
gender norms, 75, 90; and mental health,
    81–82; and therapy culture, 135–37; and
    trauma, 12–13, 55, 145, 170
GI Bill of Rights, 75–76
Goffman, Erving, 88

Graves, Robert, 62
Greatest Generation, The (Brokaw), 77
Greece, ancient, 182
Griesinger, Wilhelm, 20
Grinker, Roy, 70, 71, 72
Grob, Gerald, 83

Hacking, Ian, 15, 113
Haley, Sarah, 92, 101
Hammond, D. Corydon, 124
Harrison, Benjamin, 27
heart. *See* "irritable heart"
hereditarian perspective, 8–9, 77–78; of
    Charcot and Janet, 35, 37, 39, 40, 50,
    52; Freud's abandonment of, 41; and
    heredity vs. environment debate, 8–10,
    31, 56–57, 70, 80–81, 141–44, 168–73.
    See also predisposition
Herman, Judith, 5, 180; and recovered
    memory movement, 112, 116, 118, 119,
    131; on sexual abuse, 108, 109, 112, 114,
    209n4
Hills, H. W., 60
Hodges, Richard Manning, 32
Hoge, Charles, 156
Holocaust survivors, 89, 90, 95, 116, 128
Home from the War (Lifton), 91
Horowitz, Mardi, 102–3
Hurricane Katrina, 149, 219n60
Hyman, Steven, 180–81
hypnosis, 46, 64; Charcot on, 36–37;
    Freud on, 47–48; Janet on, 38–39; and
    recovered memory, 116, 130
hysteria, 69–70; Charcot on, 35–37,
    169; Freud on, 40–41, 42, 52; Janet
    on, 38, 39; and "railway spine," 29,
    30; and shell shock victims, 54, 78,
    198n3

Image Formation and Cognition
    (Horowitz), 102
Ingram, Paul, 122–23
International Society for Traumatic Stress
    Studies, 138
Iraq War, 2, 152–53, 154, 156–57, 158,
    220n75
"irritable heart," 24–25, 183, 193n31

Janet, Pierre, 17; on dissociation, 37,
    38–39, 112–13; Freud criticized by, 38,
    39, 196n100; hereditarian views of, 37,
    39, 40, 50, 52; hypnosis by, 38–39; on
    psychic impact of trauma, 14, 37–38,
    112–13, 169, 179
Janis, Irving, 146
Jones, Edgar, 93
Jordan, Brian, 22
Journal of Traumatic Stress, 138

Kardiner, Abram: on compensation, 97,
    176; impact of Freud on, 59, 101; on
    stressor criteria, 100–101; on trauma
    symptoms, 101, 102, 103, 176; and treat-
    ment, 63–64, 156
Kinder, John, 55, 67
King, Larry, 122
Korean War, 21, 85, 87
Kraepelin, Emil, 82
Krafft-Ebing, Richard von, 48, 111

Laing, R. D., 88
"Last Day of the Last Furlough"
    (Salinger), 76
Lembcke, Jerry, 87–88, 207n86
Lerner, Paul, 2–3, 31
liability, 176, 226n37; and PTSD, 141, 163,
    173–75; for "railway spine" injuries, 28,
    31–34. *See also* court litigation
Lifton, Robert Jay, 91, 92, 97
Lipsker, Eileen, 123–24
Loftus, Elizabeth, 131

MacKinnon, Catherine, 108
MacLeish, Kenneth, 156–57
magnetic resonance imaging (MRI), 143
magnetoencephalography (MEG), 143
malingerers. *See* cowardice and malinger-
    ing
Man in the Gray Flannel Suit (Wilson),
    76–77, 164
Marchand, Walter, 71
marijuana, 229n71
Marshall, George C., 73–74
masculinity, 12–13, 81–82, 90, 135–37
Masson, Jeffrey, 112

McFarlane, Alexander, 180
McHugh, Paul, 6, 133, 156, 178
McNally, Richard, 120, 128–29, 130,
    143, 149
memory: accuracy of recovered, 128–30;
    childhood sexual, 44, 50, 110–12, 130,
    169, 210n15; disrupted, 6; dissociated,
    37, 38–39, 112–13, 128–29; fading of,
    178, 227n43; false, 125–26, 130–32; how
    it operates, 127, 128–30, 131–32; and
    power of suggestion, 36–37, 48–49,
    50, 125–26, 133–34; psychiatry's turn
    toward, 34–35; psychic, 41, 50; PTSD
    as condition of, 30–31, 77, 166, 167;
    repressed, 39, 41–42, 43–44, 52, 127–28,
    169, 196n100; retrieval of, 129–30; trau-
    ma's relationship to, 119, 178, 227n43.
    See also recovered memory movement
Menninger, William C., 73, 80, 82–83
mental health: activism's influence on, 115;
    and gender roles, 81–82; professional-
    client relationship in, 89–90; and
    PTSD diagnosis, 104–5, 152–53; as so-
    cial concern, 79, 81
mental illness: defining, 166–68; desir-
    ability of diagnoses of, 173–78; external
    and internal causes of, 8–10, 70, 80–81,
    141–44, 168–73; hereditarian concep-
    tions of, 8–9, 35, 37, 39–40, 41, 50, 52,
    56–57, 77–78; and political agenda, 12,
    88–89; and stigma, 12–13, 24, 137, 153,
    157–58, 162, 163, 173, 186; universality
    and relativity of, 181–82
Micale, Mark, 2–3, 31, 40
Michaels, Margaret Kelly, 124–25
military psychiatrists, 79, 83, 84, 150, 157;
    on combat neuroses, 73, 141; and Viet-
    nam veterans, 91; during World War I,
    55, 73; during World War II, 70, 71–72,
    73, 84, 171
Morris, Andrew, 149
Morris, David, 137, 143, 221n89
Mott, Frederick, 170
Mrs. Dalloway (Wolff), 62
multiple personality disorder (MPD),
    113–14, 115, 120–21, 133

Münsterberg, Hugo, 127
Myers, Charles, 53–54, 60

National Center for PTSD, 155
National Co-Morbidity Survey (NCS), 144
National Institute of Mental Health
    (NIMH), 81, 180, 185, 188
National Vietnam Veterans' Readjustment
    Study (NVVRS), 150–52
"nervous shock," 30, 194n63
"neurasthenia," 24, 56, 62, 63, 167, 193n28
neuroscience, 14, 142–43, 179–80
New York Times, 21, 90, 147–48, 155
Niederland, William, 89–90
Nininger, James, 147–48

Oedipus complex, 44–45, 48
Ofshe, Richard, 123, 132
Oppenheim, Hermann, 33, 56, 178–79

Page, Herbert, 30
Patterson, Francis, 23
Patton, George, 74
Pear, Tom, 56
Peat, Harold, 55
pensions, 175; following the Civil War,
    26–27; for World War I psychic casual-
    ties, 64–67; for World War II psychic
    casualties, 75–76, 203n125. See also
    compensation
Persian Gulf War, 107, 152, 158
"physioneuroses," 63, 102, 156, 157, 167
"PIE principles," 60–61, 64, 72–73, 79
Pols, Hans, 76
popular culture, 54, 114; neuroscience in,
    179–80; PTSD in, 1–3, 137; recovered
    memory movement in, 121–22; and
    therapeutic culture, 135–37, 157–58,
    162–64, 185–86; and trauma culture,
    137–39, 151, 185; Vietnam veterans
    in, 86–87; World War II veterans in,
    76–77
Porter, Horace, 23
post-traumatic stress disorder (PTSD):
    acceptance as disease, 165–66, 186–87;
    and brain-mind relationship, 13–17, 40,

178–81; and the Civil War, 21–28; compensation for, 157–62, 174; definitions of, 4–8, 166–68, 172; and disasters, 2, 146–50, 189n5, 217n41, 218n43; *DSM* on, 7, 93–104, 139–41; external factors vs. predisposition in, 8–10, 70, 80–81, 141–44, 168–73; future of, 187–88; historical view of, 15–17, 181–82, 228n60; independence from mental health professions, 184–85; and liability, 141, 163, 173–75; as memory-related condition, 30–31, 77, 166, 167; and the military, 12, 150–62; in popular culture, 1–3, 137; and psychiatry, 3, 10, 137; publications about, 138; and "railway spine," 28–34; rates and prevalence of, 2, 53, 61–62, 69, 104–5, 150–53, 198n1; rates in combat, 53, 61–62, 69, 85, 104–5, 150–53, 198n1; and recovered memory movement, 114–15, 118–19, 134; sexual abuse as cause of, 118, 138, 145; social attitudes toward, 78, 84, 153, 184–87; stress as component of, 6–7; symptoms of, 96, 99–100, 101–4, 159–60, 167, 198n5; as term, 1–2, 229n74; therapies for, 154–56; time frame of, 89, 103, 106, 227n43; and the Veterans Administration, 2, 138, 184–85; and Vietnam War, 85–98, 150–52; and World War I, 53–67; and World War II, 67–77. *See also* "combat neurosis"; "railway spine"; "shell-shock"

post-traumatic stress disorder (PTSD) diagnosis: crusade to create, 12, 93, 167; desirability of, 10–11, 173–78; *DSM-III* on, 93–100, 101–4, 118–19; gendered differentiation of, 12–13; impact of, 104–5; symptoms as definitional criteria for, 96, 99–100, 101–4, 159–60, 167

post-Vietnam syndrome, 90–91, 95

predisposition, 101, 172–73; Charcot and Janet on, 35, 37, 39, 40, 50, 52; and debate over shell shock, 57, 170; *DSM-III* on, 98–99; vs. environmental and external factors, 8–10, 31, 56–57, 70, 80–81, 101, 141–44, 168–73; evolution of

views on, 170–71. *See also* hereditarian perspective

Prince, Morton, 113

prisoners of war, 203n126

psychiatry: antiwar, 88–93; and Charcot, 35–37; childhood trauma as focus of, 20, 42–43, 44–45, 50, 51–52, 110–12, 114, 116, 130, 169, 210n15; early study of traumatic shocks by, 5, 8–9, 50; and Freud, 39–45; on internal foundations of mental disturbance, 35, 37, 39, 40, 50, 52, 169; and Janet, 37–39; predisposition vs. environment debate in, 8–10, 70, 80–81, 141–44; and PTSD, 3, 10, 137; rise of neuroscience in, 14, 142–43; social emphasis of, 79; transformation after World War II, 71–72, 79, 82–83, 179; and trauma treatment, 45–49; turn toward memory by, 34–35. *See also* military psychiatrists

psychic memories, 41, 50

psychoanalysis, 10, 63–64, 89–90, 112, 115, 135; birth of, 40; debates within, 49, 57, 70, 89

psychological casualty rates, 104–5, 150–53; in Vietnam, 85, 104–5, 150–52; in World War I, 53, 61–62, 198n1; in World War II, 69, 104

Putnam, James Jackson, 30, 126

Railway and Other Injuries of the Nervous System (Erichsen), 28–29

"railway spine," 36–37, 174; emergence of, 11, 17, 28–31; and liability, 31–34

rape, 2, 3, 36, 99, 108, 118, 137, 171; incestuous, 108, 123; PTSD in aftermath of, 145

rap groups, 90–91, 205n44

Raphael, Beverley, 191n38

Raphael, Sally Jessie, 122

Rechtman, Richard, 163, 181

recovered memory movement (RMM), 109–18; downfall of, 125–33; and feminist politics, 115, 117, 118; and Freud, 110–12, 210n15; and Janet, 112–13; litigation against, 132–33; and mental health

recovered memory movement (*cont.*)
professionals, 109–10, 119, 120–21; and
multiple personality disorder, 113–14,
115, 120–21; origins of, 110–14; and
power of suggestion, 125–26, 133–34;
psychologists' challenging of, 126–27,
128–30; and PTSD, 114–15, 118–19, 134;
rise of, 109–10, 121–25, 134; tenets of,
114–18; and treatment, 116–18
rehabilitation programs, 66
Remembering Satan (Wright), 122–23
repression of memory: Freud's notion
of, 32, 41–42, 43–44, 52, 169, 196n100;
recovery from, 108–10; and severity,
127–28; treatment for, 46–47
Research Domain Criterion, 188
Ribot, Théodule-Armand, 34
Rieff, David, 164
Rieff, Philip, 135–36, 162
Rigler, C. T. J., 32
Rivera, Geraldo, 122, 124
Rivers, W. H. R., 57, 60
Robins, Lee, 96
robust repression, 110
Rosenberg, Charles, 94, 166, 184
Ross, Colin, 111, 127
Roth, Michael, 37, 116–17, 195n81
Russell, Diana, 108

Salinger, J. D., 76
Salmon, Thomas, 61
Sassoon, Siegfried, 62
Satel, Sally, 149
Schacter, Daniel, 127, 129, 130
Scott, Wilbur, 98
screening, 68–69, 153–54
screen memories, 44
seduction theory, 44–45, 48, 111, 112
September 11, terrorist attacks on, 147–48,
189n5
sexual abuse, 107–9; and law enforcement, 117; PTSD as result of, 118, 138,
145. *See also* childhood sexual abuse
Shatan, Chaim, 90, 92, 97, 101, 171
Shay, Jonathan, 228n60
"shell-shock," 70, 78, 191n32, 198n3; ex-

planations for, 55–59; Freud on, 57–58,
199n21; and individual predisposition,
57, 170; pensions for victims of, 64–67;
in popular culture, 62; postwar prob-
lems for victims of, 61–64; symptoms
of, 54, 62–63, 198n5, 199n11, 202n97; as
term, 53–55, 183; treatment for, 59–61,
63–64
Shephard, Ben, 61, 100–101, 146
Sherston's Progress (Sassoon), 62
Shorter, Edward, 182–83
Smith, Grafton Elliot, 56
Smith, Jack, 97, 101
social attitudes, 78, 84, 153, 184–87
Solnit, Rebecca, 146
Spiegel, Herbert, 126
Spiegel, John, 71, 72
Spielrein, Sabina, 197n109
Spitzer, Robert, 94, 96, 97–98, 102
Starr, Paul, 85, 86, 91–92
Stefancic, Jean, 138
Steinem, Gloria, 108, 111
stigma, 24, 153, 173; disappearance of,
137, 157–58, 162, 163, 186; and gender
norms, 12–13
stress, 56, 96–97, 100–101; environmental,
72, 79, 81, 83–85, 171; as PTSD compo-
nent, 6–7
Stress Response Syndromes (Horowitz),
102–3
Studies in Hysteria (Breuer and Freud),
40–42
Substance Abuse and Mental Health Services Administration, 7
suggestion, power of, 36–37, 48–49, 50,
125–26, 133–34
suicide, 26–27, 86, 138, 153
Sullivan, Harry Stack, 68
survivor guilt and syndrome, 89, 90, 101
Swank, Roy, 71
Sybil (Schreiber), 114
symptoms. *See* trauma symptoms
Szasz, Thomas, 88

talk therapies, 47–48
Taxi Driver (movie), 86

television, 2, 121–22, 137, 140, 215n16
Terr, Lenore, 109, 123, 127, 132
therapeutic culture, 135–37, 157–58,
    162–64, 185–86
therapies. *See* trauma treatment
Three Faces of Eve (Thigpen & Cleckley),
    114
transference, 47–48, 60
trauma: definitions of, 142–43, 172; exter-
    nal and environmental view of, 8–10,
    31, 56–57, 71–72, 79, 80–81, 103–4,
    106, 141–42; Freud's view of, 39–40,
    48–49, 57–59; gendered nature of, 145,
    150; memory's relationship to, 119, 178,
    227n43; neurobiological aspects of,
    180–81, 228n56; rates in general popu-
    lation, 144–45, 217n30; somatic and
    hereditary view of, 8–9, 31, 35, 37, 39,
    40, 50, 52, 77–78; as term, 4. *See also*
    post-traumatic stress disorder
Trauma and Recovery (Herman), 119, 180
trauma culture, 137–39, 151, 185
trauma symptoms: during the Civil War,
    23–26; cultural, 182–83; Kardiner on,
    101, 102, 103, 176; and PTSD defini-
    tional criteria, 96, 99–100, 101–4, 159–
    60, 167; from "railway spine," 28–29,
    30; time frame of, 89, 103, 178, 227n43;
    during World War I, 54, 62–63, 198n5,
    199n11, 202n97; during World War II,
    69–70
traumatic brain injury (TBI), 216n26
Traumatic Neuroses of War, The (Kar-
    diner), 100–101
trauma treatment: for bodily aspects, 156;
    community, 81; by Freud, 5, 45–49, 50;
    by Kardiner, 63–64, 156; and memory
    retrieval, 129–30; PTSD therapies for,
    154–56; and recovered memory move-
    ment, 116–18; for repressed memory,
    46–47; for Vietnam War veterans,
    90–92; during World War I, 59–61,
    63–64, 78–79; during World War II,
    72–74, 79
Trimble, Michael, 191n38
Tritle, Lawrence, 181

Triumph of the Therapeutic, The (Rieff),
    135–36
Trump, Donald, 1–2, 138

Unchained Memories (Terr), 123
unconscious, 34–35, 36, 51–52; Freud on,
    42–43, 50, 59
Understanding Words That Wound (Del-
    gado and Stefancic), 138
Ustinova, Yulia, 14

Vaillant, George, 104
van der Kolk, Bessel, 109, 112, 119, 155,
    156
Veteran Comes Back, The (Waller), 74–75
Veterans Administration (VA): and
    PTSD, 2, 138, 184–85; and Vietnam
    veterans, 88, 90, 92, 93, 161, 205n39
Veterans of Foreign Wars, 75–76
Vietnam Experience Study (VES), 105
Vietnam veterans: and antiwar psychia-
    try, 88–93; compensation claims by,
    158–59, 161, 177; in popular culture,
    86–87; PTSD rates among, 85, 150–52;
    response within society to, 87–88; and
    the Veterans Administration, 88, 90,
    92, 93, 161, 205n39
Vietnam Veterans Against the War
    (VVAW), 88–89, 90–92, 93, 110, 115
Vietnam War, 85–88; psychic casualty
    rates in, 85, 104–5, 150–52
violence against women, 107–9, 145. *See
    also* rape; sexual abuse

Waller, Willard, 7, 62, 64, 67, 74–75, 163
War Neuroses (Grinker and Spiegel), 72
"war neurosis," 56, 58, 66, 67, 70, 170
Watters, Ethan, 132
Wecter, Dixon, 67
Wessely, Simon, 93, 187
Wilbur, Cornelia, 113, 114, 126
Wilson, John P., 191n38
Wilson, Sloan, 76–77
Winfrey, Oprah, 122
Winter, Alison, 110, 121
Wolff, Virginia, 62

World War I, 51, 53–67; differences from
World War II, 78–79; explanations for
combat trauma during, 55–59; number
of psychic casualties in, 53, 61–62,
198n1; symptoms of psychic casualties during, 54, 62–63, 198n5, 199n11,
202n97; treatment of psychic casualties
during, 59–61, 63–64, 78–79; and veterans' postwar problems, 61–64
World War II, 67–77; attitudes toward
psychic casualties in, 73–74; differences
from World War I, 78–79; explanations
for combat trauma during, 70–72,
202n100; number of psychic casualties in, 69; psychiatric staff during,
68; psychic casualty rates in, 69, 104;
screening programs during, 68–69;
symptoms of psychic casualties during,
69–70; treatment of psychic casualties
during, 72–74, 79; veterans' psychic
damage from, 74–77
Wright, Lawrence, 122–23
Wynne, Lyman, 98

Yealland, Lewis, 60
Yehuda, Rachel, 142, 173, 180
Young, Allan, 5, 16, 145, 186